Table of Contents

The Average Rapist

According to recent FBI Uniform Crime Reports, over 100, 000 reports of rape are made annually in the US. This crime is perpetrated by average citizens daily so who is the "average" rapist? What does he look like? The answer to this question is as varied as the crime itself but there are some personality traits the average rapists all seem to share. Being aware of these traits may give the victim an edge that could well make all the difference.

On every University campus young women interact with their male counterparts on a daily basis and many coeds can tell you about the guy or the guys who seem to express anger or aggression frequently. As an average man or woman it is considered normal to express some frustration with the academic demands. Certainly the pressures of college life are understandable but in dealing with certain men who frequently exhibit hostile feelings toward their instructors or others on campus women should be on guard. These same hostile feelings can easily be translated into hostile acts especially when someone tells them "No."

Women should listen closely when men are describing women they know using words like bitch or whore and be aware that stupid or other derogatory language really means they said "No"... These men may refer to their former girlfriend in these terms or worse and condemn her for being slut. These same men often behave in a controlling manner or by being excessively jealous or possessive. Ultimately they treat their partner as their possession and through subtle threatening gestures indicate that he can do with others whatever he wants. This kind of man does not respect individual rights of other human-beings and considers women as sex objects to fulfill their own needs for gratification. This sexist attitude leads always to a rape where the man tries to make the victim feel guilty for being "uptight" and resisting his sexual overtures...

Women often want a man to accompany them to a game or dance and really don't care where they go before the event but they should because that is a good time to find out more about them. A man may intimidate in little ways in the beginning as a kind of testing the waters or it may be that he simply is that selfish. Watch out for a man that prevents you from seeing or talking to friends or family members. Keep you isolated and separated from your support network and want you to let him make all the decisions.

The personality of a rapist makes him the one who decides where to go and what to do. These decisions are his to make without asking your opinion. If this is a first date it might be wise to consider the possibility that later he may make the decision about whether to have sex with him. These personalities often want what they want and do what they want regardless of what you want. Who you will associate with and what you both will do should be a decision you both agree on.

.

What's next?

Here are a few things to keep in mind if you are assaulted, and may be helpful to tell a friend who has been assaulted. First of all rape is a criminal act and the victim is not at fault. Second the victim is still alive and now can do something about this crime just as she would do if a thief stole her purse with her paycheck and credit cards. Just as in that theft she has been robbed and she needs to get to a safe place as fast as possible so someone else will not take advantage of the situation. Finally for the crime of rape you can choose to report it to the police or not. Just like when a thief has robbed you of your money you know people will believe you because why would you rob yourself? There are people who will believe you and who can help. It was not your fault!

The whole purpose for writing this book is to get women of all ages to get medical attention as soon as possible to make sure you are physically well. In addition to the emotional and psychological trauma experienced during and after a rape, survivors often must deal with physical trauma. A rape is a violent act and involves bruising, cuts, and even broken bones. Most rape victims suffer internal trauma such as the tearing or bruising of the labia, vaginal wall or damage to the urethra.

There are critical concerns regarding disease. Rape involves the mucus membranes and disease can be transmitted easily. If for no other reason than this women must seek medical care. These diseases can often be effectively treated immediately after exposure through a series of antibiotics but once the disease is firmly entrenched the problems are greatly magnified. Sexually transmitted infections (chlamydia, gonorrhea, and the human papiliovirus can lead to cancer and death. HIV is a devastating disease and the drugs necessary to keep it at bay are both costly and have side effects. Get to the clinic or hospital and cooperate with the procedures contained in the Rape Kit if for no other reason than to save you the fear of not knowing and the suffering of not having known.

After an assault, it can be very difficult to feel safe and to return to your normal life. Many survivors go through a normal progression of shock, psychological distress, and attempts to forget and feel normal. Some people call this Rape Trauma Syndrome (Hyperlink). If you are experiencing symptoms of Rape Trauma Syndrome, you may want to seek support. There are many places you can turn: Family, friends, significant others

Under the Violence Against Women and Department of Justice Reauthorization Act of 2005, access to the rape kit is provided without qualifications. The law reads that states may not

"require a victim of sexual assault to participate in the criminal justice system or cooperate with law enforcement in order to be provided with a forensic medical exam, reimbursement for charges incurred on account of such an exam, or both."

Under this law, a state must ensure that victims have access to an exam free of charge or with a full reimburscmcnt, cven if the victim decides not to cooperate with law enforcement investigators.

The importance of this law in the understanding of the crime of rape and the understanding of the magnitude of the problem cannot be ignored. Only 100,000 rapes were reported to U.S. law enforcement agencies and represent a small part of the actual rapes of all types taking place. Government estimates find that anywhere from three to ten rapes are committed for every one rape reported. And while rapes by strangers are still underreported, rapes by acquaintances are the most under reported. Yet, based on intake statistics at various rape counseling centers the numbers are far higher.

Anyone can be a rapist. Statistics show that most victims are assaulted by someone they know, an acquaintance, family member, friend, dating partner or spouse. It may be hard to believe that you could be hurt by someone you know. Remember that rapists and abusers are manipulative and deceitful. They are adept at creating situations where they can take advantage of a person's trust and good will. Studies have shown that there are some people who are more likely to be sexually aggressive than others.

Watch out for people that do not listen to you, ignore what you say, talk over you or pretend not to hear you. Rapists have little respect for their victims and tend to ignore your personal space boundaries. These men want to dominate by standing or walking too close or attempt to touch you without permission.

To the law, courts and police it appears as if the rape was not serious enough or that the victim invented the rape if she does not report to the medical facility preferably within an hour. Also washing and douching destroys evidence (sperm, saliva, blood, skin, and hair, etc.) that is used to identify the rapist and to apprehend him. Therefore, it is crucial that immediately or as soon as possible after the rape that an examination of the victim is recorded in a well-documented, detailed report.

Upon arrival at the rape clinic or hospital, a trained nurse meets the victim at the emergency room. Injuries are extensive as in the case of a 65-year-old woman with broken pelvis and concussion, an adolescent victim of gang rape suffering from vaginal and internal hemorrhaging. Or the five-year-old with multiple stab wounds, the physician on call will provide the necessary emergency services. Registration formalities may be done in a closed examination room. If the patient cannot understand written and spoken English, arrangements will be made for an appropriate interpreter. The nurse will explain briefly the necessary procedures and obtain the alleged victim's written consent for the physical examination, photographs if indicated, collection of specimens and ancillary evidence such as clothing, and the release of such information to proper authorities.

Injuries must be assessed and they can range from bruises and cuts to traumatic as in the case of a 65-

year-old woman with broken pelvis and concussion, an adolescent victim of gang rape suffering from vaginal and internal hemorrhaging. There have even been attempts to murder the victim as in the five-year-old with multiple stab wounds; in all these cases the physician on call in the ER will provide the necessary emergency services.

It is important to note that not all private physicians can be relied upon to treat rape victims—even family doctors—as they do not generally wish to become involved in court appearances or feel they cannot afford time away from their other patients. Furthermore, some hospitals and private clinics, for legal or other insurance reasons, will not treat a victim but will transfer her to another facility where suitable treatment may be obtained. If this is the case, the alleged rape victim will be given initial care and after an assessment of the trauma the nurse or physician will offer a tactful and humane explanation of her referral to another better equipped hospital.

For the most part, procedure is standardized, and the medical team is trained to maintain a chain or evidence in cooperation with legal authorities' requirements. If the victim is to be referred, medical personnel handle her as minimally as possible but certain types of evidence such as possessions with blood, urine, semen, saliva, etc., stains are allowed to dry if possible, and then placed in separate paper bags; these bags are then put in plastic for transporting with the victim.

The victim may encounter this when she seeks treatment at an outpatient or school health clinic. Often these facilities do not have the trained personnel or the jurisdiction to handle a rape case. The nurse notifies the receiving hospital of the referral of the alleged rape victim and sends a copy of the emergency room treatment form with the victim. The alleged victim will be requested to carry it with her and present it to the receiving nurse. If the police or county authorities have been called in, they may accompany her to the other hospital.

It is important to understand that the hospital staff are trained to maintain the chain of evidence and the victim should cooperate with the process and not bathe, shower, brush your teeth, or go to the bathroom until after the exam. This is important for preserving evidence. If possible, do not change your clothes. If you already have, put your clothes in a clean paper bag, such as a grocery store bag, and bring them with you to the emergency room. If possible, go to a SANE hospital first. There is a medical hotline to inform the victim of the nearest SANE unit or the 911 dispatcher can provide that information.

Without a medical report that meets the legal system's requirements, no case can stand up in court. Instead the rapist will continue to pursue his criminal activities undiscouraged and undaunted by either the woman he assaulted or the society he, the victim and all of us must continue to live in. Even if he is arrested without evidence he will be released. Rape will go unpunished and the statistics will continue to soar.

More women and children will be hurt and exploited and more and more men will be encouraged to rape.

The Rape Kit and Exam

The sexual assault forensic exam kit (commonly referred to as a "rape kit") is the collection of DNA and other forensic evidence, which is kept by the SEXUAL ASSAULT NURSE EXAMINER OR A SEXUAL ASSAULT FORENSIC EXAMINER nurse or medical provider until it is sent to or picked up by law enforcement or the crime lab. The rape kit is stored until the victim determines whether or not to pursue a case.

The kit is generally a large envelope or cardboard box, which can safely store evidence collected from your body or clothing. While the contents of a sexual assault forensic exam may vary by state and even by jurisdiction, it may include items, such as: - Instructions-Bags and sheets for evidence collection-Swabs-Comb- the Kit has 16 separate steps to collect evidence. There are detailed instructions for each step that the provider should follow.

These specimens include collection of blood, urine, hair and other body secretion samples, photographs of injuries (such as bruises, cuts and scraped skin), collection of clothing (especially undergarments). Envelopes for hair and fibers and documentation forms

A "Jane Doe Rape Kit" enables a victim to have forensic evidence collected without revealing identifying information. Each Kit has a unique number assigned to it. All evidence collected will be placed in envelopes or bags and labeled with this number. The victim is given a code number they can use to identify themselves if they choose to report the crime at a later date. Victims are now allowed more time to decide whether to pursue their case, a decision that can be difficult to make at the time of the attack. Just remember that the storage and retention of evidence collection kits vary and may not match the statute of limitations.

The victim has a right to choose whether or not to prosecute and may also decide what parts of the exam she will allow to be completed. Victims have the right to accept or decline any or all parts of the exam but it is Important to remember that critical evidence cannot be presented at trial if it is not collected or analyzed.

Some victims have reported that their kit was not analyzed in a timely manner and women's group's protests to police crime labs have been effective in ending the delay, a phenomenon known as the "backlog". This backlog is due partly to the fact that even though all rape kits are brought to the Crime Lab these kits are only analyzed when the survivor makes a report to police and the processing takes time.

Another consideration is that treatment at a medical facility must be obtained within a reasonable timeframe after the assault. To be valid the rape kit must contain evidence of treatment at a hospital within 120 hours of an assault. The police report may not be made at the time of the assault for a number of reasons but the rape kit if done in time will be analyzed once the report is filed and the rape kit results available for presentation at the trial.

It is important to understand that Each Kit has a unique number assigned to it. All evidence collected will be placed inside envelopes or bags and sealed these are then labeled with this same identifying number. The victim will receive a copy of this number and should give it to her attorney if seeking civil damages as well as criminal prosecution.

The Exam

A forensic medical exam may be performed at a hospital or other healthcare facility, by a sexual assault nurse examiner (SEXUAL ASSAULT NURSE EXAMINER OR A SEXUAL ASSAULT FORENSIC EXAMINER), or another medical professional. This exam is complex and on average, takes 3-4 hours.

While this may seem lengthy, medical and forensic exams are comprehensive because the victim deserves and needs special attention to ensure that they are medically safe and protected. In addition, it is important to collect evidence so that if the victim chooses to report the crime to the police, they can access the stored evidence.

The medical record itself documents all the specifics of the physical examination and the patient's medical history. It will record what specimens have been obtained as well as the patient's care. The medical record of a rape victim is preserved in the usual confidential manner as for any hospital patient, and the results of the examination, tests, and medical specimens, will be released to the appropriate law enforcement agencies upon, and only upon the consent and request of the patient.

After the hospital staff obtains written consent. The alleged victim is then referred to as "M.E. case" (Medical Examiner's case) or simply "patient." The attendant nurse records the condition of the patient's attire;

photographs may be taken, then she will help the patient remove her clothing and slip, into the white hospital gown. The nurse will see that the articles of clothing are dried before bagging and then bagged separately in paper bags. Care will be taken with the undergarments so that pubic hair does not fall out or other possible foreign bodies lost.

To start, the medical professional will write down the victim's detailed history. This sets a clear picture of existing health status, including any medications being taken and preexisting conditions unrelated to the assault. The patient's medical history, taken by the nurse or physician, includes a brief general history with regard to past illnesses, drug allergy, surgery and other pertinent information, a gynecological history, record previous gynecological surgery, contraceptive method if any, existing or possibility of existed or suspected pregnancy, past coital history, history or possibility of past gynecological infection, questions of possible medico legal import as to whether she has changed clothes, douched or bathed since the alleged rape, and time of last previous coitus, if any, and the number of assailants.

The physician will ask carefully phrased questions to help evaluate the patient's psychological state, and to find out if there are underlying mental disturbances which could be exacerbated by the alleged rape. The nurse may ask the time of the last sexual intercourse, which might seem irrelevant; however, if the patient was raped only a few hours after voluntary exposure, the sperm must be typed in order to identify the source.

After recording the patient's medical history, the physician proceeds with the physical examination in the presence of a nurse or attendant; and if the patient requests an additional witness to be present, such as a friend, family member. This will be permitted. If the patient has requested a social worker or counselor to be present, they will assist her just as the nurse assists the physician.

Next there is a head-to-toe, detailed examination and assessment of the entire body (including internal examination). The physical examination includes a complete description of any injuries like bruises and/or lacerations with special reference to injuries that may have been incurred during the attack. Examination of the head, face, and neck are important for it is this area, which often incurs the most damage. The eyes are particularly vulnerable. Damage to the trachea and larynx due to being choked or forced fellatio, as well as fissures of the skull and vertebrae may require the assistance of neurological equipment and trained personnel. Torso, arms and legs are inspected, for they are often subjected to bruising from a variety of blows made by fists or weapons like guns and steel pipes. All of the above fall under the classification of general appearances and photographs will be taken as corroborative evidence.

The physician's and attendant's next concern is to help the patient lay on her back on the examining table, and get her feet in the stirrups, as in a routine pelvic exam. The nurse usually tries to calm the victim as she is gently pulling the white gown apart. At this point the victim may seem frustrated or confused, wondering what more her body must be made to endure. She generally has many questions and needs reassurance and support to understand what is happening.

Often the physician or nurse explains the medical procedures but many have several patients to treat and must rely on staff or a counselor to answer questions. The rape crisis social worker or SEXUAL ASSAULT NURSE EXAMINER OR A SEXUAL ASSAULT FORENSIC EXAMINER is also a trained counselor. The SEXUAL ASSAULT NURSE EXAMINER OR A SEXUAL ASSAULT FORENSIC EXAMINER nurse is aware of the many aspects of rape from hospital to courts. She can explain the process from the first encounter with the police to the reactions of family and social pressures. She will stand by the patient's head during the examination, rendering female emotional support and critical medical information when needed.

I am encouraged to see female physicians stepping forward to handle rape victims in both emergency rooms and during long-term gynecological care. I think this makes the victim trust the physician, knowing that because she is a woman she is more involved, more sensitive. The female ER or OBGYN can put the experience into perspective and can lessen the trauma of insensitive men or women whose behavior has ranged from joking to a cold and even critical attitude, which only serves to magnify the victim's trauma. Under the impact of feminist ideas, this condition has improved, yet many women still complain about a lack of sensitivity from male and female friends.

Many victims suffer internal injuries to the genitalia, such as bruises, lacerations, and contusions to the pereum, hymen, vulva, vagina, cervix and anus, are carefully examined. This is done with a in the vagina which slowly dilates the vaginal canal. First the physician describes the condition of the vagina and cervix and notes carefully any lacerations, hematomas, presence of foreign bodies, etc. In the case of the child rape, the difference in size between an adult female and small girl must be taken into account; medical treatment for the child victim will be adapted to the little girl's size; special small examining instruments will be used and lacerations will be repaired under general anesthesia.

During this part of the examination, the patient may hear the doctor remark something about getting a "good specimen," or as the nurse hands a slide to the physician, the patient may watch—curious, a little guarded perhaps—as the specimens are then taken: a swab from the vaginal pool to detect the presence of semen, another from the vulva. Wet smears of the vaginal pool fluid, and oral or rectal secretions, will be immediately examined for evidence of sperm, specifically for the presence, condition and motility.

Two slides of these secretions are placed in Pap fixative for pathology in the determination of prostates acid phosphates. If this cannot be done promptly, the slide will be refrigerated, as the enzyme deteriorates at room temperature. This is especially important in the case of coitus with vasectomies male. The physician must then take two permanent, dried smears on clear glass. These can be examined for blood group antigen and precipitant tests against human sperm and blood. Additional specimens of secretions may also be taken for the same purpose— endocervical (rectal and or pharyngeal, if appropriate) culture for gonococci and a urine sample for pregnancy test if indicated.

Other physical specimens are taken in addition to the above. Pubic combings will be made by the nurse and placed in a labeled bag. Twelve or fifteen of the patient's pubic hairs are cut as close to the skin as possible and are put in a separate labeled bag to be submitted with the combings. Scrapings from under the nail beds are taken, separately bagged and labeled. This is done if there is a possibility of recovering the alleged assailant's skin, which can be used as evidence in a court of law.

The physician or nurse shall never transfer specimens to an unidentified messenger or technician. Whenever possible they will transfer the specimens directly to the pathologist or to the appropriate police representatives. If any specimens cannot be transferred at once, they will be locked in a secure place and transmitted directly to the pathologist in the morning.

Specimens may be kept refrigerated if held for a period of time. These will be placed in a container sealed with evidence, tape or with clear plastic tape sealed over the identification date. The identification includes the patient's name and number, name of the person obtaining the specimens and that person's name, title, address, date and hour of collection and transfer of specimens. Any bullets or foreign bodies found will also be clearly identified and maintained with other specimens for a minimum of 48 hours by the facility, in a secure locked area. This care is necessary so that the chain of evidence may be maintained— the hospital can be held responsible if it is not.

Venereal disease is one of the hazards of rape and either the doctor or nurse will speak about treatment for sexually transmitted infections (STIs). Depending on the circumstances of the rape and the possibility that the victim may have been exposed during the assault the treatment will vary. Both the hospital and the state have specific protocols for how the victim may receive prophylaxis as well as any referrals for needed follow-up counseling, community resources and medical care and the doctor will discuss the various methods of prophylactic treatment. Often the physician will suggest an antibiotic dosage known to be effective in aborting incubating strains of syphilis and gonorrhea as a precaution.

Rape victims for a time after the assault may suffer from vaginitis, a vaginal infection that is the result of antibiotic therapy disturbing colonies of bacteria normal to the vagina and allowing a foreign strain to multiply. Vaginitis is identifiable by the following symptoms: discharge, localized rash, and burning sensation when urinating. In time, the normal bacteria recolonize; yet, some infections assume a chronic condition, which can be both an irritating and painful reminder of the assault.

In large cities and on University campuses women have in great numbers become more aware of their human rights, the pressure of their numbers reporting their rapes to medical facilities has made it necessary for hospitals to organize rape programs in conjunction with legal requirements. Because sex can now be a choice for women, we are coming to realize that the only way to reach our respective goals is by recognizing ourselves as people first, with the authentic human feelings of courage, fear, aggressiveness, passivity, love and hate—in short the entire range of human emotion.

Date Rape

Women raped by men they know--acquaintance rape--is not an aberrant quirk of male-female relations. If you are a woman, your risk of being raped by someone you know is *four times greater* than your risk of being raped by a stranger. Those rapes are happening in a social environment in which sexual aggression occurs regularly. Indeed, less than half the college women questioned in the Ms. survey reported that they had experienced no sexual victimization in their lives thus far (the average age of respondents was 21). Many had experienced more than one episode of unwanted sexual touching, coercion, attempted rape, or rape. Using the data collected in the "social life" on America's college campuses:

A University survey of 6,159 college students enrolled at 32 institutions in the U.S. found the following: · 54% of the women surveyed had been the victims of some form of sexual abuse; more than one in four college-aged women had been the victim of rape or attempted rape; · 57% of the assaults occurred on dates; · 73% of the assailants and 55% of the victims had used alcohol or other drugs prior to the assault; · 25% of the men surveyed admitted some degree of sexually aggressive behavior; · 42% of the victims told no one.

Over the years, other researchers have documented the phenomenon of acquaintance rape. 25 percent of the undergraduate women surveyed had at least one experience of forced intercourse and that 93 percent of those episodes involved acquaintances. Almost 29 percent of women surveyed reported being physically or psychologically forced to have sexual intercourse. A survey of male college students: · 35% anonymously admitted that, under certain circumstances, they would commit rape if they believed they could get away with it · One in 12 admitted to committing acts that met the legal definitions of rape, and 84% of men who committed rape did not label it as rape

For a case of rape to be recognized in the courts, a number of contributing factors must first be considered by the state's attorney. The determining factors rest on the evidence and on the states attorney's discretion in filing the charge of rape. Theoretically an elected official's decisions must coincide with the law and the attitudes of the individuals in the state or community based on their traditional racial, political, religious and economic values.

Date rape is now commonly referred to as "acquaintance rape." First-hand accounts by women who have been raped by men whom they knew provide a background for analyzing this crime. These stories are meant to make women aware of how this type of rape happens, how to avoid the pitfalls of certain situations, and how to acknowledge that a rape has taken place even if the person is familiar. The statistics indicate that this is a widespread occurrence often ignored by women who deny what happened or feel they won't be believed. This book will enlighten young women about what constitutes an assault against them and how to deal with it.

This is true in every state, community and even country but we are presently discussing attitudes and beliefs held by the wider consensus in the American culture. Rape, when it crosses the racial barrier, becomes problematic and specifically if the woman is a Black, Hispanic or Oriental and the man a Caucasian. Unless there is a known pattern or serial assault record for the perpetrator the case seldom reaches a courtroom. Although rape is a common crime to women and children in all of these racial or ethnic groups, the number of actual cases tried reflects the American media-programmed view rather than the actual statistics.

In acquaintance rape, the rapist and victim may know each other casually--having met through a common activity, mutual friend, at a party, as neighbors, as students in the same class, at work, on a blind date, or while traveling. Or they may have a closer relationship--as steady dates or former sexual partners. Statistics show that a full 70 to 80 percent of all rape crimes are acquaintance rapes. Although largely a hidden phenomenon because it's the least reported type of rape (and rape, in general, is the most underreported crime against a person),

There have been a number of surveys in the last 30 years on American campuses which indicate patterns of behavior that are consistent such as the fact that 90%

of rape victims attending colleges and universities knew the offenders. - *Bureau of Justice Statistics, The Sexual Victimization of College Women, 2000.* This same study reveals that 48.8% of college women who were victims of attacks that met a study's definition of rape did not consider what happened to them rape.

Based on first-person accounts, studies and data from a nationwide survey of college campuses conducted by Ms. Magazine devastating portrait of men who rape women they know. · 43% of college-aged men admitted to using coercive behavior to have sex, including ignoring a woman's protest, using physical aggression, and forcing intercourse. · 15% acknowledged they had committed acquaintance rape; 11% acknowledged using physical restraints to force a woman to have sex.

The Ms. survey reveals that 25% of the college women polled have been the victims of rape or attempted rape, 84% of the victims were acquainted with the attacker and 57% of the rapes happened on dates. One in 12 of the male respondents admitted to acts that meet the legal definition of rape or attempted rape many organizations, counselors, and social researchers agree that acquaintance rape is the most prevalent rape crime today.

Many young women on college campuses refuse to talk about their rape. Other victims mention their feelings as "being in a state of shock" or talk of the "unreal" aspect of the rape crisis. Adult women react differently to rape according to their psychic makeup and the circumstances of the assault, but the primary reaction for almost all women is anger and fear. When the victim's true feelings are unbearable, she may try to psychologically sublimate one feeling and substitute it with another. She may seem calm and composed, at time she be controlling or hiding her true feelings behind a quavering smile of resignation.

After the initial shock the traumatized victim may be unable to stop crying or may exhibit other visible signs of emotional distress such as uncontrollable nervous shaking or extreme fear unable to speak and dry mouth.

When rape is suspected the appropriate response is to suggest a medical exam as soon as possible. The friend or family member is not trained to handle certain responses to this crisis but must rely on the society to provide suitable care and qualified caregivers. University health centers are often closed at night except for emergencies and many do not have a SANE nurse on call. It may be necessary to drive to a hospital ER for treatment.

Once the victim arrives at a hospital she should be aware that she is in control of the entire exam. Before each step of the Kit, the medical provider will explain the step and ask her if she wants to continue the exam. Most rape victims need care and are physically abused. Physical trauma includes soreness and bruising but can be far more serious and be classified as attempts at murder. Peers too often dismiss this aspect of rape but the statistics show that the threat of death is involved far more than many would believe. State laws provide for specific charges and punishment for forced sex acts such as sodomy. It is a crime and a physical injury that results in a great deal of discomfort in and around the mucus membrane. Other symptoms physically related to the rape are vaginal discharge, vaginal itching, and burning sensation during urination and vaginal infections.

The reverse is also true: many psychological problems are manifested in physical ailments and appear on the surface as various neurotic symptoms. Of these we could include tension headaches, fatigue, and disturbance of sleep patterns, stomach pains, and loss of appetite, nausea, and general discomfort. In the case of gang rape, when a woman is forced into repeated coital acts or simultaneous rectal and vaginal mountings, traumatic tearing of soft tissues supporting structures that separate vagina, bladder and rectum may cause the victim to react later to sexual intercourse by an involuntary constriction of the lower one-third of the vagina (disparmeia). Unfortunately the result of not seeking immediate medical and psychological care only serves to deepen the crisis of rape.

Date Rape Drugs

If the victim finds it difficult to talk about the incident or is unresponsive when asked to recount it she may have been drugged. The memory of events may be fuzzy or the location is confused, the victim is not certain what happened or if anything happened. When questioned she may have difficulty recalling anything but will experience haunting dreams or flashbacks due to the effects of a date rape drug.

Women must understand that certain drugs can and are used to make victims incapable of resisting the attack or remembering the incident altogether. In 1996 the federal government passed a law called the Drug-Induced Rape Prevention and Punishment Act of 1996. This law makes it a felony to give an unsuspecting person a date rape drug with the intent of committing violence, including rape, against him or her.

If the man encourages a woman to drink beyond her tolerance level or wait to make a sexual advance until she is extremely intoxicated then this is a rape. Alcohol is the #1 date rape drug. Unfortunately, the law does not eliminate the use of alcohol as a relaxer but it is a rape situation when a woman is being encouraged to drink heavily. A man can quickly become a "mean drunk" who becomes aggressive, angry, or violent if he is rejected.

It is illegal to give a person a date rape drug or a sedating drug of any kind with the intention of having sexual intercourse with that person. If the victim or medical provider at the time of the rape exam suspects that a drug or drugs were used in connection with the assault then a blood and/or urine sample may be collected as a part of the exam. This sample is then tested for drugs and is another part of the exam. The samples are included in the "Toxicology Kit" and will be tested for the presence of drugs and alcohol in the blood of the victim.

Substances can remain in the blood stream for up to 96 hours after they were ingested so testing beyond this timeframe may not provide valuable evidence to present at trial. In addition many substances leave the body in less than 96 hours so a negative result does not mean that the victim was not drugged. Testimony from eyewitnesses as to the victim's state of mind may indicate the use of a date rape drug even though the chemical was not present at the time of the Kit collection.

Prescriptions, over the counter medications, alcohol and recreational drugs will also be detected with the test. This can be a factor in pursing criminal charges. If the victim chooses to complete a Toxicology Kit and the findings indicate the presence of controlled substances she may not want to prosecute.

The victim may fear that this evidence will lead to charges filed against them even before the trial and may back out. If controlled substances are a factor at all the victim may decide not to even report the assault to the police. The victim who does decide to pursue prosecution must understand that the toxicology results may also be given to the perpetrator as part of the legal process.

The Toxicology results will generally be available after 12 weeks so the victim has time to make a decision. If the victim reported the assault to police and a toxicology kit was completed the results can be obtained from the Certified Sexual Assault Investigator in the town where the assault occurred or the District Attorney handling their case. Women should be aware that there are prescription and banned drugs used by predators. The best defense is awareness of their names, uses, and dangers so here is the list and the information you need to know.

Ketamine

Street Name Special K, Vitamin K, Ket, Kit Kat,

Ketamine, is ketamine hydrochloride, used as an animal tranquilizer and an anesthetic. It is legal only under a doctor's supervision. Special K has been used as a date rape drug.

Ketamine comes in a white powder, tablet, or liquid. The powder form can be added to tobacco or marijuana to be smoked. When Ketamine is taken orally the effects begin within 10 to 20 minutes and 5 to 10 when snorted. Effects can last up to 48 hours.

Kit Kat is a harmful drug that acts as a dissociative anesthetic that impacts the central nervous system by separating perception and sensation. Ketamine has some very obvious symptoms and causes impaired attention, and memory loss. In high doses and or if the person is sensitive to the drug there may be bouts of delirium, fear to the point of paranoia.

Kit Kat causes slurred speech, breathing problems and sleepiness to being unconscious during the assault. One characteristic that makes it attractive to sexual predators is its effects of amnesia, bizarre hallucinations, and compliant dissociation.

Rohypnol

Street Name Roofies, Rope, Ruffies, R2, Ruffles, Roche, Forget-pill, Mexican Valium

Rohypnol is a sedative. Ruffies depress the central nervous system and act like a sleeping pill. This drug is prescribed as a pre-anesthetic in Europe. Rope like Special K causes amnesia, a lack of resistance and slower of psychomotor responses. Rohypnol takes effect quickly after ingestion - about 10 to 30 minutes. Effects of disinhibition and amnesia can last from 8-24 hours. Rohypnol is not FDA approved as a sedative-like Valium and is manufactured in Mexico and South America and transported illegally into the United States. President Bill Clinton signed a bill in 1996 that made using or selling Rohypnol a federal crime.

Ruffies are small white pills, which are in packs marked Roche (the name of the manufacturer F. Hoffmann-LaRoche Ltd.), Because of its amnesiac characteristics, sexual predators often use Rope because its effects are intensified when combined with alcohol. The pills dissolve in liquids with no odor, color, or taste so it is impossible to detect. Roche, the manufacturer, has produced a pill that dissolves more slowly and turns a drink blue. The drug is detectable in the blood for 24-60 hours after ingestion.

Many victims have reported that after Rohypnol was slipped into their drinks, they blacked out and woke up unsure of what had happened. Unfortunately the loss of memory does not mean a loss of consciousness blurring the lines of consent. Victims can be appear alert and capable of making decisions at the time such as agreeing to leave the party or going to an apartment but still experience complete memory loss of the what happened. The loss of memory may prevent people from reporting the crime soon enough to be tested for the drug. Higher doses or combined with alcohol may produce drowsiness, confusion, dizziness, hot flashes or cold feelings and intestinal problems.

GHB

Street Name Liquid Ecstasy, G, Grievous Bodily Harm, Georgia Home Boy, Scoop, Easy Lay

GHB is odorless, colorless, and slightly salty tasting liquid. Ecstacy is virtually undetectable once it is dissolved in a mixed drink. Any strong flavorful drink like a margarita can mask its slightly salty taste. GHB affects brain chemistry by increasing levels of dopamine, is a brain chemical involved with motivation, pleasure, initiation, and control of movement. GHB enhances sensitivity to touch and reduces inhibitions.

Easy Lay can act like a sleeping pill because it can deepen REM sleep and also as an anesthetic. The FDA banned Ecstacy from legal sale in the United States in 1991. This illegal street drug was banned in 1991 when 57 cases of GHB poisoning were reported by the Center for Disease Control. GHB can be lethal when taken with alcohol and the dose is unregulated due to the manufacturing of this dangerous drug by basement chemists.

Scoop causes incoherence, dizziness and severe headaches that can lead to seizure and coma. GHB is manufactured in basements with primitive equipment and cheap chemical components by amateurs or college students with limited understanding of complex drug compounds effects on the human body. This fact only makes the drug more dangerous and unpredictable.

Lower level doses of GHB can produce amnesia and muscle weakness which also makes the issue of consent or resistance compromised. Since it is impossible to determine the concentration or purity of this drug or the potency when combined with alcohol or other depressants, it can be fatal. Since GHB depresses the central nervous system it can lead to unconsciousness, respiratory arrest, and death. According to the Drug Enforcement Agency, both deaths and thousands of overdoses have been recorded.

Many women have been exposed to this drug in unknown concentrations without their knowledge and consent. As the drug of choice for sexual predators Easy Lay is as it's street name implies easy to slip into someone's drink as a date rape drug. Scoop is absorbed into the body quickly and takes effect within 15 minutes. Taken alone the drug's effects can last between 2-3 hours but in combination with alcohol, the effects may last from 20-30 hours. It can knock victims out, leaving them defenseless against rape. In addition, GHB is undetectable in the urine after 12 hours.

Alcohol

The number one date rape drug isn't GHB, Roofies, or Ketamine. The number one date rape drug is alcohol. When on a date where liquor is served here are some safety tips that have worked for other women. First of all never accept an open drink from a stranger. Only drink from containers you have opened yourself. If you are at a party or dance remember to never leave your drink unattended, just the guy you are with. If you must leave the table and ditch the drink, get a fresh one. If you think you have been drugged get your cell phone and call 911 immediately or get someone to take you to the hospital

Go to parties with close friends, if you leave a party tell a friend where you are going and with whom. Keep a close watch of what others are doing and how you are feeling. Date rape drugs work quickly and intensively. If your friend seems more intoxicated than what the amount of alcohol would warrant. Get them home and get help. If you feel more intoxicated than what the amount of consumed alcohol would warrant you may have been drugged. Immediately leave the table and call 911 or tell a trusted friend to take you to the hospital. Tell your friend that you are feeling sick. Get medical attention...

These substances can be identified and can remain in the blood stream for up to 96 hours after they were ingested. Toxicology results will generally be available after 12 weeks and victims who reported the assault to police can get the Toxicology results from the Certified

Sexual Assault Investigator in the town where the assault occurred or from the office of the District Attorney handling their case.

If the victim or medical provider suspects that a drug was used to facilitate an assault, a blood and/or urine sample may be collected as a part of the rape exam. If the victim thinks she may have been drugged, she can ask that a Toxicology Kit be collected. The samples in the Kit will be tested for the presence of chemical substances, such as date rape or street drugs and blood levels of alcohol.

A negative result does not mean that a victim was not drugged only that a chemical was not present at the time of the Kit collection. Prescriptions, over the counter medications, alcohol and recreational drugs will usually be detected with the test. If you choose to complete a Toxicology Kit and report the assault to the police, you should be aware that the toxicology results may be made available to the perpetrator as part of the legal process.

College age women may use recreational drugs or may take prescription drugs for stress or a previous emotional condition and this should not interfere with the legal process for most rape cases. Remember the rape exam does not require the victim to prosecute it only provides her with the knowledge and evidence that if she chooses to do so she can. Unfortunately the presence of drugs in her body may be considered an offense unless there are indications that the lack of consent extended to the use of these drugs.

Women with promising career paths and high academic achievement give various reasons for not going back to school after an assault and may drop out for a semester or two. This is one of the many detrimental aspects of the aftermath of rape and how it interferes with a woman's rights. The constant tension contributes to disruption or termination of a great deal of social interaction with peer groups especially with coed activities. The victim withdraws from scheduled activities with other young women and men in their school, church or community. This is especially true when the assault was by another student at the same institution.

Some young women can alleviate these anxieties about returning to the classroom by changing schools; others try to change campuses within the University system or curricula. Rape has such a devastating effect on self-image and a young woman's developing professional ego that a few simply withdraw altogether. Rape is so demoralizing to the young psyche that even an honor student will have a declining academic record afterward. While every young woman should determine her own aspirations and goals, it is very hard for her to know how high she really could go if the traumatic experience of rape interferes with the opportunity of advancement that an education offers.

Recovery from Rape

Rape is one kind of crisis experience, just like the death of a loved one, a natural disaster or the termination of a relationship through divorce. Although the victim may be very badly hurt from the experience, she will survive and overcome it as the others are doing, but the recovery will be slow and it will have many stages. Immediately afterward the victim may experience shock or disbelief, and a flood of feelings associated with the event.

Although every survivor you encounter will be unique, many will have one thing in common: Rape Trauma Syndrome a cluster of emotional responses to the extreme stress experienced by the survivor during the sexual assault. More specifically, RTS is a response to the profound fear of death that almost all survivors experience during the assault. RTS occurs in two phases:

Initial Reaction

The initial response to rape is shock and can lasts anywhere from a few days to a few weeks after the attack and is characterized by Post Traumatic Stress Disorder (PTSD) is a clinical diagnosis often ascribed to people who have experienced extreme or prolonged exposure to stress such as physical/emotional/sexual abuse, violence, war, natural disasters etc. Symptoms of PTSD include depression, sleep disturbances, flashbacks, or erratic mood swings and are particular emotional and physical effects of rape.

The rape experience has the effect of disrupting the lives of many victims and their families. Many victims were fearful for their very lives, and the trauma of that experience can last for months or years during which even a small incident can lead to a flashback and to responding to the fear of death just as they had experienced. The victim of rape may display any of a number of emotional responses from uncontrollable sobbing to shouting or cursing. At the other end of the spectrum they may laugh nervously, talk incessantly about superficial things as though to reconnect with a calmer existence or seem catatonic.

Friends or family should be prepared for these displays of emotions and should respond reassuringly to the victim who appears to be agitated and talks a lot. Sometimes the support person will find themselves acting in a similar manner at the same time. This responding in concert is appropriate and can be reassuring and reaffirming to the victim and allows her to get it "out" in her own way of responding.

Some victims of rape do everything in their power to contain their emotions while inside they are raging. The victim may appear to be sitting calmly during the Police interview and may respond to questions in a detached, seemingly logical manner. Inside emotions of fear, sadness bordering on a kind of grief or feelings of disgust and anger. This is a response to the crisis of rape and is just a few of the different ways of dealing with rape.

In the initial response phase the victim will be in shock and exhibit disbelief. They may appear to go numb refusing to acknowledge the rape while their minds and emotions are trying to comprehend the recent events and to process the emotions associated with the experience. The victim of acquaintance or date rape may have a very difficult time overcoming the shock. If the assault was especially brutal or a date rape drug was used the victim may completely block out the assault.

Following the shock and disbelief most survivors experience other emotions or mood swings. They may feel that they are lucky to be alive if the attack was brutal or violent and if they have sustained severe injuries. Some women who hold traditional beliefs may feel humiliated while certain religious beliefs may reinforce feelings of being defiled or degraded. All of these responses, as well as the many that are not listed, are a part of the person's values and the societal expectations within their cultural or ethnic orientation. In short, whatever the victim experiences within the context of their beliefs is to be respected.

The survivor will probably notice a disruption in usual sleeping and eating patterns. They may not be able to eat or sleep, or may eat more than usual and be unable to stay awake. They may report nightmares in which the survivor relives the assault. These may evolve into dreams in which the survivor takes the violent role in some way, in effect reclaiming the control lost during the assault. Although both types of dreams may upset them, dreams are part of the healing process.

Adjustment Phase

During the adjustment phase the victim makes every effort to get her life back after the sexual assault. This phase is characterized by the victim relearning how to cope with everyday activities without the debilitating after effects on their lives after a sexual assault. Much of their success or failure can be attributed to the coping mechanisms they have developed and already possess and significantly are impacted by whether or not they successfully have coped with severe trauma in the past.

The behaviors which led to the rape are important to consider because this is a prime time to face a drinking or drug problem and get help. Rape occurring within a relationship or marriage can precipitate a divorce or break-up and can lead to a host of other emotions. Some victims were raped because of or in conjunction with their ongoing emotional or psychological problems. The most successful career executive can be overwhelmed and their emotions which were under control prior to the assault may be unleashed by the trauma of the assault. Long buried fears or hatreds may surface especially if the victim was assaulted previously, especially within the last two years.

Victims may have difficulty returning to pre-assault social patterns. They may feel an increased distrust toward others in general and an increased suspicion of men in particular. They may have a shorter temper, or easily break into tears. Some reactions may be the result of a specific component of the assault. For example, if the survivor was assaulted while alone, they may want to be with other people constantly. If they were gang-assaulted, they may withdraw socially and rely on a few significant others for companionship and support. The survivor's social patterns after the assault may depend less upon the conditions of the assault and more upon the survivor's personality. Many survivors feel a strong need to "get away." They may visit parents. They may move, especially if they were assaulted at home. They may change jobs or leave school. All these actions are "normal" in that they represent what the survivor needs to do in order to regain control over life.

Denial of the effects of the assault, or of the assault itself, is a common reaction during the reorganization phase. Denial may be a component of the survivors' recovery, since it gives them space to catch their breath before beginning the stressful task of processing and resolving the trauma. Denial that lasts longer than a few hours or days, however, is detrimental to their recovery.

Depression, guilt, and a general loss of self-esteem are all common psychological reactions. These symptoms suggest that they have turned their anger inward, and that they have unresolved fears. Remind them that they are in no way responsible for the assault and that nothing they did could ever justify the violence they have experienced. Encourage them to direct these negative feelings toward the assailant and away from themselves.

The survivor may experience phobic reactions to stimuli that remind them of the assault or their assailant. Phobic reactions are extreme manifestations of anxiety. For example, if survivors were assaulted outdoors, they may be afraid to leave the house. If the assailant had alcohol on his breath, this odor may remind survivors of the assault and make them nauseous. They may experience a general paranoia, or panic attacks.

The assault may disrupt the sexual life of the survivor because sex, which usually involves pleasure, was instead used as a weapon to humiliate, control and punish. It will probably take some time for the survivor to disassociate the sexual assault from consensual sex. Acts the assailant forced that the survivor was not used to doing will probably cause particular difficulty. Survivors may experience physical pain during sex, have difficulty relaxing, or be generally indifferent to sex. At the other extreme, they may desire sex all the time. Most likely, their behavior will fall between these two extremes. If the survivor was a virgin at the time of the assault, they may have a heightened fear of their first consensual sexual encounter.

Survivors may be concerned about their partner's reaction to them after an assault. They may wonder if their partner will feel differently toward them. Because of the range of stresses the survivor experiences after an assault, consensual sexual relationships and other friendships can be placed under heavy strain. Current statistics indicate that about half of all survivors lose their love relationships within a year of sexual assault.

The survivor may report continuing gynecological/genital problems. If they were physically beaten, the survivor may continue to experience pain. Sexually transmitted diseases can be a further concern, as well as pregnancy. Nightmares may also continue. If nightmares continue in a manner that makes them lose sleep or that fills their waking hours, they might want to consider counseling.

Tech, Sext and Rape

The Internet, cell phone, iPad and tablet PCs are all technological innovations that influence our lives in the twenty first century. These in innovations contribute to the generation gap and the disparity between rich and poor becomes even more apparent. The manipulation by pornographic or sexist images of men acting out frustrations with violence encourages rape by portraying sexual expression in the context of violence as the last avenue open for individual freedom.

This freedom of expression within the context of violence is considered the male prerogative against institutional elitism and the encroaching technocratic reorganization of society. Women are the expendable products to be consumed in the exercise of this "expression". Changing legal codes and greater citizen participation in socio-political decision making can effect change within the broad tenets of the Constitution and the Bill of Rights. Lawful protest sooner or later is reflected in social and legal issues.

Women have equal abilities to contribute to a technological society and equally possess the fundamental adult capabilities necessary to effect change. All citizens can function more fully as active participants in a changing society. Women can, by exploring the flexibility of our legal codes and adapting the law to the needs of the times, change the society and its norms; but change and adaptation come from within as well as without.

The image of crime in the cinema and on television combined with crime reports, newspapers and on the radio form a picture of a violent society, a society in which laws are circumvented or openly violated as a normal part of that society. Of all the media's outlets, television carries the messages to the most people. Violence and violent related activities dominate the mass media, an integral involvement with the destruction of personal property in various dramatic demonstrations in which psychological intimidation is used to define social relations.

The media exercises a considerable amount of power in shaping the value orientation of the society as well as cultural orientation through the manipulation of goods and services displayed within the context of these dramatic presentations. Media role models and their attitudes in the cinema portray the changing ethics of a society and exaggerate a motivating force for power as one achieved through violence and sexual exploitation.

Media technology employs experts— psychologists whose living consists of toying with human weakness by exploiting ego-burdened adults whose desires and conflicts are repeatedly paralleled to infantile material needs. This manipulative psychology is not only thwarting to the individual's development of whole person identity, but to realization of society's goals toward 'liberty and justice for all,"

Your Job and Rape

The circumstances of the rape may also contribute to a disruption in the victim's career or occupational lifestyle. Some young women who planned to finish college before marriage drop out for a while and find that the emotional aftermath of rape is too much. They may try other careers or pursuits and never return. After the victim has dropped out of school she may need to find a job often in today's difficult job market and without the skills and diploma she had planned on having before entering the job market.

Employment either before or after the rape is never easy and the victim may find her stress coping skills are affected as well. Even if she relocates or finds a good job unless she resolves the issues that could have been addressed at the time through the professional services offered in conjunction with the rape exam she may fail. The victim may continue to respond in an inappropriate manner to the slightest suggestive comment or gesture from a coworker and suddenly quit or change jobs within a short time period following the assault.

Many previously competent employees fall behind in their workload and are forced to quit work if the rape was by a male coworker. Their sudden departure is much to the dismay of their coworkers who are unaware of the rape. The company is faced with recruiting and training a replacement on short notice and the victim is faced with the difficulties of finding new employment, putting physical, if not mental distance between themselves and their assailants. Others are fearful that the assailant might seek revenge and feel they are forced to quit and even to change their address.

Victims of coworker rape express the opinion that they must make these decisions regarding employment and housing in order to regain a sense of security and independence. This is why counseling is so vital and only a trained SANE professional can put things in perspective. Without medical care and support the victim is torn between what she considers to be her coworkers with whom she confides opinions and not real solid advice.

Educators, employers and families should accept this attempt by the rape victim to outwardly "adjust" by helping her honestly re-evaluate her life-style and encouraging her to make only the necessary changes. The victim's post-rape physical condition will have an important effect on her psychological wellbeing and may be the determining factor. Whatever the victim feels she needs to do to become a secure individual should be encouraged as long as she has taken the time to consider all of her options. She should only make those decisions when it is absolutely mandatory to her psychological readjustment.

Women are usually concerned about the possibility of pregnancy resulting from rape, in post-menopausal women, preventive treatment is rarely recommended, nor to women who are currently on oral contraceptive pills, using an intrauterine device or surgically sterilized but a medical checkup is critical. A drug approved for prevention of unwanted pregnancies by the FDA is commonly known as the "morning after" and pill may be prescribed at the time of the exam. The social worker or counselor will provide a follow up phone call to remind the victim of any further recommended treatments or tests. Since victims often sublimate the entire rape experience, they are likely to forget future medical tests.

A distinct pattern of sexual behavior develops as a result of rape, which is clearly discernible by comparing previous sexual activity to the trauma of the forced sexual acts and the victim's resultant loss of libido. The woman feels anxiety at the prospect of any sexual encounter. Many women express concern over future relationships, especially those involving men as sex partners. Women who were free and open sexually with men suddenly cease to experience orgasm. In addition, the victim often enumerates sexual losses, dwelling on former engagements and other breakups in her life—the accompanying worry and uncertainty contributing to a self-perpetuating cycle of frigidity.

Although husbands can be a major source of support because they are more in touch with the victim's feelings her needs and her strengths rape and its effects on parenting has yet to be fully understood but many women are aware of how their own rape has affected their children and how it has changed their life-style. Women who have assistance in childcare between these impairments and the resultant stages in the family life cycle overcome psychological trauma sooner than those who do not. Even simple tasks usually performed by the woman such as marketing, cooking meals are overwhelming.

The moral and physical responsibility for the care of children in the family requires the assistance of their husbands or other family members—mother, sister, or aunt. It is not uncommon for victims to move to a family member's home for a few days or a week so that this assistance can be more easily obtained. Without help, this woman falls into an emotional depression that may span several months. As time goes on the unfriendly attitude of the rape victim toward herself and her husband or family increases to contempt. The rape victim wishes to act aggressively; she does so first by exhibiting hostility in sex and as her avenues of escape are frustrated, she may express the wish to die.

Suicide attempts are calls for help and are the result of frustrations of the rape victim's conflicts among family, friends, or in the society. Suicide is a common threat in all ages of women who have been victims of rape. Immediate medical care and reinforcement of positive activity in dealing with the rape crisis lessens the possibility that the victim will attempt to take her own life. Without trained counseling or the physical care and emotional support of a knowledgeable professional suicide becomes the tangible means of expressing the rape victim's pain.

Women feel instinctively that the sexual act should represent a commitment of the persons engaging in the act to each other, accompanied by love and shared lives, Unearthing the true natures of ourselves as women today is healing to the victims of rape because it gives them a better perspective of the society and allows them to function freely as total persons within it. Women seeking to correct the imbalance of women's position in society through their personal lives are part of an overall healing process.

Adolescence and Rape

Adolescence is a difficult enough period without complications of rape. It is important for parents to consider the sexual development of a child before their own personal psychological motivations. Due to a child's rapidly changing body and maturing ego-consciousness they may be self-conscious, shy, or lacking in self-confidence despite any semblance of extroversive behavior. Peer-group approval and the consequent worry about self-image can make the adolescent appear moody and unpredictable.

In a survey of high school students, 56% of the girls and 76% of the boys believed forced sex was acceptable under some circumstances. - A survey of 11-to-14 year-olds found· 51% of the boys and 41% of the girls said forced sex was acceptable if the boy, "spent a lot of money" on the girl; · 31% of the boys and 32% of the girls said it was acceptable for a man to rape a woman with past sexual experience; · 87% of boys and 79% of girls said sexual assault was acceptable if the man and the woman were married; · 65% of the boys and 47% of the girls said it was acceptable for a boy to rape a girl if they had been dating for more than six months. –

Young women can be trusting of their boyfriends as they are of their friends and may not understand what is happening before it is too late. Many parents are confronted with the problem of a lack of knowledge of self-defense. If the victim doesn't fight back, perhaps it's not rape. This mistaken belief is part of a wider belief system of how men and women should interact.

The truth is when a young woman is being forced to have sex, she may believe that the rapist is capable of other types of violence and she may fear that she could be killed or injured. The young victim may be in shock of what is happening. She may also decide that it is too late to fight and that will only anger the rapist. The victim may have been coerced into having sex, or may have been forced to have sex while intoxicated or impaired by a date rape drug.

What effects does rape have on a young girl or teenager? The signs of emotional trauma, which the teenage victim exhibits, range from crying to shaking or a general restlessness and wanting to be alone. This reaction is not unusual in rape victims but then neither is hysteria. We now have to think in terms of a devastating blow to a developing psyche. Studies have shown that anyone who deals with a young teenager in crisis must be sure that they communicate their support for the victim.

The best way of initiating this support is immediately after the assault to seek medical care at a clinic or hospital equipped and staffed to handle the trauma of rape. Usually, the survivor will report a general soreness throughout the body. They will also report pain in the specific areas of the body that were targeted during the assault. These specific pains may be the result of actual physical trauma, or may be a psychosomatic response. At the time of her exam the victim will receive the care and support she needs in the first hours after and attack. She will be treated with a respect for her personal privacy and even if she hesitates to go out of being helped against her will she will thank the person who took her there.

Intense emotional outbursts are common in this age group and when combined with the trauma of rape the emotional stress suffered by a teen-ager may be immense. Some young people, on the other hand, have severe emotional problems that the rape only exacerbates. Troubled teens have little resistance due to drugged states of consciousness, and then we are dealing with significant, psychologically damaging characteristics of rape. Criminal networks prey on runaway youths who are drugged and then forced into prostitution. The statistics in some cities represent a national problem.

An adolescent girl may feel alone or hostile and that she can only share with someone she is romantically involved with and may think others are insensitive to her fears. When a child is left to try to sort things out without counseling they may become restless, rebellious and defiant, all behaviors indicating that these youngsters have great difficulty in adjusting to a situation which is so detrimental to their mental health. Again these behaviors do not go unnoticed and all too often the report is filed by one or more teachers who recognize these problems associated with changes in emotional status as they begin to surface in the classroom.

This powerful message of forced sexual activity and rape is in direct conflict with her learning response in school where she is superior to the boys. Immediately her perspective of male female interactions is altered and certain classrooms or activities may present considerable stress and difficulty. Without an abundance of expressed love, patience and guidance (non-authoritarian), the cognitive process can be blocked and her female personality development greatly impaired.

A young victim's educational pattern need not suffer if she receives medical and psychological care on an ongoing basis and follow up counseling through her school and church. The child's innate cooperative spirit and competitive desire to better herself in sports or extracurricular activities should be encouraged and the one bad experience will be put into perspective. Withdrawal from reality is a major problem in the young who have been the victim of rape and it is even more apparent in the tense and uncertain aftermath.

The girl thinks that she alone must decide whether to talk about it and may avoid seeking medical attention. She may need medical help and hesitates because she does not know anything about what will happen if she does go to a hospital. How often have we heard "You wouldn't understand? It is at this moment that the supportive person takes the initiative tells her in no uncertain terms that she needs medical care. Just two words in a calm but firm voice, "Try me".

The victim needs to have a strong system of friends and family for emotional support and these close associations can determine how well the victim recovers from an assault. Family and friends must first of all treat the victim with empathy and the victim must be able to trust them and understand that they can go to them as needed. This show of understanding and strength will make the difference at that moment and perhaps for the rest of her life. Be firm but not pushing and it could be the beginning of trust; once trust enters a relationship then the emotions held in check by some teenage victims come out. Offering immediate understanding and support are crucial to a teenager's psychological coping and healing. Too much emphasis has been on the physiological aspects of teen rape when it is the psychological aspects that are far more damaging and long lasting.

Many rapes go unreported and resultant injuries are hidden under makeup. Disease or pregnancy is blamed on the victim by her parents or friends. In many cases she may have been threatened by the assailant either by verbal or physical assault during or after the rape and her fears of his retaliation if she tells anyone will cause her to withhold information and not seek the medical and psychological care she needs. Women with a history of rape or attempted rape during adolescence often do not have this support system and are almost twice as likely to experience a sexual assault a second time. These women are also three times as likely to be victimized by their husband.

The opposite reaction of apparent gaiety, perhaps laughter has been observed—some victims can't stop this irrational behavior. These girls become risk takers and are often seen doing crazy things or just "wild". Others withdraw and pretend to be engrossed and playing a game on their cell phone or computer to avoid detection of their emotional state. The teen will seem to be texting half of the school when in reality she is desperately reaching out for reassurance that she is normal. Others refuse to talk for fear of conveying too much about the boy who could not help himself to protect him from punishment for the rape.

Teens will not disclose how they really feel to the school nurse, counselor or someone they are not deeply involved with, or to an authority figure that they think is insensitive to them. This is where the training of a SANE nurse can make a difference and radically change the young victim's perspective on the assault. In both withdrawal and exuberance their behaviors are blamed on anything but the rape. Without proper care the teen will put up a superficial façade but the reality is the adolescent victim now lives in a private world of fear.

Many young victims flee reality through sleeping and often come right home from school and go to bed. Many victims experience dreams and nightmares, which are part of the mind's long-term readjustment process. While some girls are able to discuss their reoccurring nightmares others are not. It is not unusual for the younger victim to scream in the middle of the night and refuse to talk about it the next day. Pushing her to discuss the nightmare without considering the possibility that her fear may be based in the real world will lead to further confusion and disorientation.

Rape can result in emotions running so strong that the victim may have a nervous breakdown, particularly for young girls in the large cities where complex and impersonal junior and senior high school institutions allow her to get lost in the numbers. She may begin to retreat after an assault and become withdrawn. A pregnant girl may be forced into welfare dependency and depending on her age coerced into an arranged, early marriage. Yet the statistics on the failure of early marriages are sobering since at least three out of five teen-agers who marry after getting pregnant are divorced within six years.

Pregnancy is a possible outcome of rape for a teen and depending on the circumstances may also result from the attempted rape of a young girl just past puberty. The medical precautions necessary to prevent it will force the parents of an adolescent to recognize their daughter's sexuality. In fact some parents may feel more distress over the issue of sexuality than the rape, particularly if they have not previously talked to their daughter and allowed the school to educate the child. There are times when parents may have avoided talking about it for a specific reason and that reason may lead to the perpetrator.

Almost all psychological problems associated with rape originate in the victim's attempt to gain personal control while under a circumstance, family or society in which she feels she has little control. Guilt and self-blame combined with this feeling of helplessness have been directly related to attempts at suicide. Pregnancy or the fear of pregnancy from rape has also been the determining factor in many attempted suicides of adolescents, some of which were passed off as "accidents* Not all teenage girls slash their wrists or swallow sleeping pills; some just go on a dietary roller coaster.

The SANE professional, after completing the necessary medical care, may recommend group therapy and teen group's encounters. Within the intimate sphere of the family a teen's sex-role identity is developed and many family values offer the young teen an equal opportunity for gaining personal identity within that emotional, intellectual and sexual interaction. Sex between spouses should be loving, respectful and cooperative. The family relationships that embrace this can become a richer and more fulfilling life experience. The discovery that other families share similar problems: she is less alone. Although rape may not be talked about it is still very real and painful for millions of individual teenagers throughout America.

Older Women and Rape

Women feel instinctively that the sexual act should represent a commitment of the persons engaging in the act to each other. Many older victims have had a long term marital relationship accompanied by love and shared lives and are unprepared for the realities of rape. Their experience of sex within marriage may have been considered a duty but exercise in mutual body respect and accompanied by pleasurable consent. Older women may still desire a sexual partnership but in the case of rape they have been denied a total human relationship.

Rape can be extremely damaging psychologically to the elderly, to widows or single women living alone. Sometimes there may be no one for the aging victim to turn; or, there may be a husband in his seventies, for instance, who when told of the rape may become a coronary patient. If the woman is beginning to feel less sound physically, she may be particularly concerned with the close encounter she had with violence coupled with her concern over the event as a sexual assault. It is crucial that the counselor and members of the consciousness group do not overlook the sexual issue, as many women are still sexually active at this age.

Older women sometimes hold beliefs that are part of a societal view that has radically altered over the course of forty years. One common misconception is that it is apparent by their appearance who is a sex offender. The truth is that men who rape come from all walks of life and ethnic backgrounds. Rapists can be anyone from a new friend, distant relative, minor acquaintance or even a complete stranger who offers to help. Rapists may be clean cut and may even be good looking, a Christian man which they use to make their approach to older victims easier.

Older women are portrayed by day time soap operas as the old maid or divorced women forever 50 and looking for a man. The media sex typing of plunging neckline and somewhat easy demeanor does not include many women and those who do not conform to this image are limited in box office productions. The female villain is more likely to exhibit such traits as lying or conspiring and when confronted they show an inherent stubbornness and foolishness that leads them into impossible situations.

Older women have been accused of falsely claiming rape to get even with a man with whom they once had a crush on or with whom they once had a relationship. Nationwide surveys of police departments indicate rape is one of the least falsely reported crimes, reporting a rate of 2%. Rape is also one of the most underreported crimes, with only 1 in every 10 assaults being reported to the police. Older women are the least likely to falsely report any crime and are the most likely to not report at all.

After an assault rape victims of all ages develop certain fears and phobias specifically related to the location of the attack. These fears are common seen in the elderly victim who may fear being alone if the attack occurred in the home or conversely many older women will stay close to home if the rape occurred outside her house. If the rapist was a stranger she may exhibit irrational fears of crowds or of being followed by someone.

Loving family members strive day and night to give the elderly victim the support and understanding she needs yet they often lack the training or knowledge to make the critical difference in healing. Only by encouraging her positive viewpoints and helping her to develop her physical wellbeing will psychological improvement become apparent. Other older women who have experienced the aftermath of rape, whether personally, or through family or friends can be a valuable source of support. The victim's friends should get involved and not merely an impersonal show but with genuine feeling to end the single older woman's cycle of alienation.

Especially for an older victim nurses and doctors are not merely an impersonal professional performing a routine job but sincerely try to address all of the older victim's concerns. They can be a source of valuable information or they can find someone who does. The SANE nurse understands the healing process and is sincere; they are truly a case of women helping women. These caring nurses can make a difference by offering the single older victim support, letting her know that they are there for her, by their own desire to help.

The resuming of previous activities and putting the experience into perspective with respect to her entire life, is more complex. The victim will have a lot of decisions to make on her own, but all of them will be healing and will ultimately lead to resolution of the event. It is important to remember that throughout the entire process the older adult victim alone must come to her own conclusions about the rape and the role of the friend or family member is not one of crusade but of one of support It is in her new relationship to the rest of humanity that the "victimized" woman can "open up" and view her own creativity, then her innermost spiritual aspect can approach the problems of readjustment.

This constitutes the final phase, the resolution of the event at which time the individual has really dealt with her emotional feelings about the assault, understands her options and can make informed decisions of how life will progress from here on. At this point, these women may be said to have completed the process, gone full circle. Having overcome the fear and the hurt, now armed with a greater faith in themselves as persons, they have conquered what few people have ever mastered— themselves.

.

Children and Rape

Small Children do not usually understand rape as a sexual act but relate to it in terms of pain or fear. Often a very young victim is silent or unresponsive. This is not because she does not experience emotional trauma because she does not have the vocabulary to voice her feelings.

Sex crimes are crimes of passion or desire is a myth that crumbles in the aftermath of the rape of a small child. If nothing else the rape of a child proves beyond all shadow of a doubt that rape is a crime of violence,

power and control. The adult male rapist often use objects for penetration of small children. Their bruised and mutilated bodies have clearly offered the rapist little sexual gratification.

Pedophiles have been portrayed as men who molest and rape children and teens in order to get sex when nothing could be further from the truth. The real gratification for a Pedophile comes from intimidating, humiliating, and degrading their victims.

Young girls in early adolescence have been portrayed by the media and the defense attorneys as responsible for the assault and as having provoked the sexual assault by the "sexy" outfit they were wearing when the rape occurred. Youth and fashion have little to do with the crime of rape as a thorough analysis of what a child was wearing is documented in the rape exam and proves that fashion is not a determining factor for children who have become victims of sexual assaults.

Parents should show serious concern when listening to the child's report of "alleged" rape. Very young victims often begin bed-wetting accompanied by nightmares or insomnia. Frequent complaints of stomach ache or severe headache or pain in an arm or leg may result from the assault or can be physical manifestation of the child's psychological trauma. Others are expressing themselves by giggling, fidgeting, avoidance or suddenly crying. If you have ever seen a small child who has been raped or if the child is your own you can quickly distinguish the truth of the situation. Even if it isn't rape it may still be molestation, and she should be urged to talk about it.

First is the need for medical care and the child should be taken to a medical facility for evaluation. Without a medical report that meets the legal system's requirements, no case can stand up in court against rape. Instead the rapist will continue to pursue his criminal activities undiscouraged and undaunted by either the child he assaulted or the society he, the victim and all of us must continue to live in. Even if he is arrested without evidence he may be released. Rape of a child will go unpunished and the statistics will continue to soar. More children will be hurt and exploited and more and more pedophiles will be encouraged to rape.

Once at the hospital the parents will be requested to give permission before any examination and treatment may proceed. If the parents or legal guardian cannot be located and the child is brought by another family member then the Office of the States' Attorney will be contacted.

The small child can sometimes give the nurse a verbal account of the assault. This will help the nurse identify injuries and tell her where to look for evidence on the small child's body. A physical exam may be performed to assess, document, and treat injuries that are not immediately apparent and to locate other bruises, lacerations, and injuries to head or possibly fractured bones.

The SANE nurse may collect samples from the small child's mouth, vaginal and/or anal cavities, fingernails, and other parts of the body that the perpetrator touched during the assault in order to collect DNA specimens. In addition the SANE nurse must ask the small child if he or she played with anyone in the past 5 days who may also have left behind DNA. This step helps law enforcement determine which DNA was left by a playmate and which DNA belongs to the perpetrator. If there are any indications that the child was drugged a toxicology kit may be completed and blood and urine samples collected.

To induce the young victim's response, the nurse or doctor will ask questions concerning her physical wellbeing, for example: How are you feeling? Do you hurt anywhere? If so, where? These are good questions to remember because they are useful to expose important information about the attack and these types of questions should be tied to her emotional state. The questions asked are as follows: Does this pain frighten you? How does this cut or bruise make you feel? If the child is too upset or completely withdrawn, the SANE nurse will encourage her to discuss the events of the day, starting with what happened at breakfast, school, etc., bringing her gradually closer to the area of sensitivity—the assault. Get her to tell the story or "secret".

When the child is in a calmer state she often can relate the events in story fashion, remembering otherwise lost details and even little bits of information from which to build a description of her assailant or assailants. This will take time because the child's mind cannot process the events because she has no field of reference for the attack. Once the full story of the rape is out, her mind can begin to sort through the event and cope with what she feels. Children learn to identify events in their lives much the same way as when learning to read. Time increases the child's ability to comprehend and in time and with parental understanding she can overcome most of the negative societal expectations.

The Department of Children and Family Services must also be notified by telephone and a report will be made. Parents are sometimes reluctant to sign the release papers particularly if incest is suspected. In these difficult circumstances children are dependent on the willingness of their parents or mother to report the crime committed by the close relative or the father.

Even other adults or relatives who may be aware of the criminal offense are reluctant to become involved.

Whether rape or sexual molestation has occurred is important in the medical diagnosis; therefore, only hospital personnel will take the incidents relevant to medical treatment. All other statements surrounding the incident are of an investigative nature and should be entrusted to law enforcement agencies.

Sometimes the young victim, due to medical circumstances, has not been interviewed by the police, or cannot be interviewed then the SANE nurse will ask the critical questions needed for proper care. Understanding the circumstances can sometimes benefit the physician and a social worker or another member of the emergency room receiving personnel may obtain this information. This information is confidential but when a crime has been committed it is considered evidence.

The evidence the police need to know is primarily the location of the alleged offense—building, house and geographical area, etc., —description of any involved vehicle, name of the alleged offender, description of alleged offender, description of what occurred, time of alleged rape, names of any potential witnesses if known should be recorded. This information (taken by adding consultation forms to the hospital record and carefully written to avoid misinterpretation), along with the medical record and the hospital staff responsible may be used in the investigation or become evidence for the state in a court of law.

In cases involving child molestation and incest the first consideration must be to those children under ten-years-of-age. The unfortunate child is most likely to have been abused by someone she knows and she may be reluctant to go to her own family for support. This situation is indeed difficult and not for an untrained person to handle. The emotional trauma may be extreme particularly in young children who may have no sense of what has happened and the adult may send the wrong message causing increased trauma.

Parents and other family members should seek medical care for the child if there is obvious physical evidence, i.e., bleeding and bruises about the genital area, other signs of abuse. More subtle signs include a young child's vague story of someone putting his hands under her skirt; the sudden avoidance of a parent, relative or close friend of the family, an abrupt decline of interest or achievement in school. Attempts by the family to hide incest almost always result in another person such as a neighbor or teacher reporting a suspicion of sexual abuse.

Outward signs of distress are manifested in a child who will only sit and stare, crying occasionally and fidget for no reason. If the child is silent, unresponsive and refuses to answer the questions asked by the doctor, by the police, then parents or the mother may have threatened her by her attacker.

Negative psychological effects in the child victim are sometimes caused by parental anxiety and over-reaction than from the molestation by a family member, which the child generally perceives differently than adults do.

A common reaction to stranger molestation is an enhanced protectiveness of both parents in their continual reinforcement that the child should not trust anyone. While it is easy to become over-protective of one's child after this experience, most professionals advise to instead make every effort to return the family to a normal life-style.

The need for human interaction is never more crucial than when the crisis of rape affects a child. Children must continually be taught to interact and to relate to people around them and this leads to a confused relationship status. After an assault by a teacher, coach or church member parents or other supportive persons must now encourage their child to return to their previous school activities.

A supportive parent should never interrogate, but rather listen, support, and comfort. One must never give the child the impression that it was their fault that they were touched or sexually abused. Absolutely the child must never in any way feel responsible for the assault. Adults must allow the child to discuss the incident in as much detail as possible and only a SANE trained professional can get to the truth with the least trauma to the young victim.

Families are not trained or emotionally equipped to handle molestation or incest. Parents of children, who have suffered molestation, should give their child the benefit of contact with a trained counselor when the parents feel they are unable to handle whatever situation has arisen. Depending on the parent's education level the question of responsibility for the rape shifts from the victim to the family to the rapist and back to the victim again. The supportive parent will avoid lashing out with "You're a troublemaker, a liar," or "How could you embarrass us like this—the family name". The child's ability to cope with the abuse depends a great deal on the way the incident is handled by adults as opposed to any television soap opera's interpretation.

Parents are also victims of the psychologically damaging experience of their daughter's rape and attempt to "blame someone," which they usually narrow down to themselves the molester or sometimes the child for being disobedient. Sometimes there is an organized effort by the father and brothers of the girl to find the molester. The emotional distress suffered by the family members at the discovery of the sexual assault may prove to be too much for the child's fragile psyche. Parents are faced with the difficult task of not imposing conservative or traditional sexist values expressed in terms like "violated," or "lost her innocence".

Some parents blame themselves for the incident and worry that they did not supervise the child adequately or were somehow negligent. This "blaming themselves" is a common guilt reaction immediately after and in the weeks following the assault. The entire family's self-esteem is lowered as parents and close relatives often appear anxious and fearful of the impact on the child's personality. Occasionally this concern is voiced as angry blame toward the child, compounding the child's confusion and feelings of guilt. The child is reprimanded repeatedly: "Never get into anybody's car" or the speech ends with the phrase, "You knew better" This negative approach makes the child aware of her parents condemnation and lack of emotional support and could induce permanent emotional scars.

Many parents decide that their daughter should not return to grade school immediately as a means of protecting her from further trauma; consequently after the rape, the child misses an average of two to five days. Excuses for this interruption in routine range from medical or legal appointments to various physical or emotional problems. When the child does return, the parents may become overly protective, a condition which is also disturbing to the child. These parents are continually reinforcing never to trust anyone and behaving like bodyguards when escorting their children to and from school.

Clinical case studies prove that children who are sexually exploited are often less creative and less expressive of themselves and grow increasingly more so as time goes on without immediate professional care. The very young child is often completely overwhelmed by the rape experience; they retreat, they become emotionally disturbed, exhibiting symptoms similar to an adult victim such as difficulty sleeping, loss of appetite, and extreme bouts of emotion.

During the first seven to ten years of schoolgirls outperform boys by a significant margin. This higher achievement pattern is due to a genetic difference; earlier physiological maturity allows girls to achieve better than boys in every academic area during the elementary school years. The predator many times exhibits an immature child psyche and misreads the girl's behavior as responsiveness. These individuals may have been victimized as a child and never received professional care while others are serial rapists. To the early adolescent aged victim the rape or molestation experience conveys that she is lesser than the male, that she is subordinate to him in a humiliating, demeaning way.

Children will often identify with television or movie characters or even actual people sports heroes or Nobel Prize winners with whom they consider to be their ideals. If given the education they will learn to be their own judge of how to respond to threatening situations and under proper supervision will make the right decisions that will decrease the probability of another bad experience. Sadly if the child is not given the medical care and emotional support by trained professionals in the aftermath of rape then the negative "instant replays" may occur again within a short period of time.

Incest and Families

Social workers across the country told me that women react with shock to the fact of their husband's incest. Incest is seen as the family's entire way of life is under siege. The mother's fear of physical injury to herself and/or her other children, or fear of losing her husband either through abandonment or imprisonment, forces her into a silent condoning of his behavior, in general, the mother has little control over the situation. Distraught, she may herself abuse the child by slapping her, or if her daughter is older she may "throw her out of their house.

These negative reactions are not confined to low-income families; those more financially well off seek psychiatric help—ironically not for the father who has committed the crime. But for the daughter, the "victim" there may be few options. Since child molestation and rape are usually the culmination of a serious psychopathology existing in the family or one of its members, psychiatrists go -> to great lengths to determine the girl's "eagerness" to participate in the illicit sexual activity. Furthermore, many mothers feel justified in this approach stating that they felt forced to compete with the daughter for their husband's attention.

Through listening to victims cope with their rape the trauma that very young children are experiencing have been established. Each individual reacts differently to the crisis of rape, but age is always a determining factor. What is the psychological effect of a premature sexual encounter on a minor? When it is not a matter of rape, but sexual molestation, children and young girls are often accused of lying. This is particularly true in cases of incest. I have witnessed the frustrations of young girls when they finally get the courage to tell their parents or mother and then find that they don't believe them or that the mother sides with the father.

If the assailant is someone she has been taught to love and respect, such as her father, the girl suffers from doubts; stunned and in shock she may also feel guilt about her participation. She thinks that surely she must be the "bad girl" and that is why her father became so angry when she told her mother* obviously the rejection of those close to her can cause very deep psychological injury.

This rejection coupled with the girl's feelings of guilt is often too enormous for her to accommodate and serious emotional damage to the point of schizophrenia may result. The victim may exhibit behavior ranging from extremely passive and fearful to wildness on some occasions or riotous on others. Overall there is a great tendency to emotional involvement and withdrawal and to exhibit ambivalent affection. Younger victims evidenced hyperactivity, intense sibling rivalry, and several overt symptoms such as enuresis and school problems.

This condition rarely improves with time; sadly, the trauma deepens as the young victim grows old enough to understand what happened, or as the older one contemplates her family situation. For the most part, the incest victim's reactions are dependent upon her behavioral conditioning by her mother or the torment may go on for years as some ease are not reported until the daughter becomes pregnant by her father. Unwanted pregnancy added to the impact of fear, anxiety, shame and loss of self-esteem can severely retard the adolescent's emotional development.

Pregnancy

If for some reason a young woman discovers that she is pregnant and needs an abortion she should be aware of some facts relating to abortion, which I will cover here in a summary fashion. Understanding care is offered at the abortion clinics and their staff is highly responsive to the patient's treatment as a whole person with emotional as well as medical needs. Will usually visit the clinic three times; besides the actual abortion, there are generally two outpatient visits: a pre abortion medical work-up and a post abortion follow-up.

Up to the twelfth week of pregnancy an abortion can be done quickly. The whole procedure takes about five to ten minutes, with little blood loss, minimal anesthetic and a low risk of complications. The operation may be performed in a doctor's office or in an outpatient clinic. First the physician conducts an internal examination to verify the pregnancy and check the angle of the uterus. A speculum holds the walls of the vagina apart throughout the operation. Next a uterine sound is passed through the cervical canal into the uterus to ensure that the canal is not blocked, and to estimate the measurements of the uterus. A local anesthetic injection is sufficient to stop pain.

After the abortion, some cramps and fainting can occur if she gets up too quickly from the operating table. A woman will have period-like bleeding for a day to a week afterwards. She must not douche after an abortion because the cervix remains slightly dilated and a douche can force fluid into the uterine cavity. For cases between the twelfth and fifteenth week of pregnancy an abortion usually it takes about ten to fifteen minutes. The work-up for a D. & C. is the same as that for uterine aspiration, including pelvic examination, after a local anesthetic injection and cervical dilation the abortion is performed. Once the canal is dilated the physician inserts a curette into the cavity of the uterus with an ovum forceps and gently scrapes away the placental membrane. There is greater blood loss and recuperation is slightly longer than that for uterine aspiration.

Infection after a properly performed abortion is fairly simple to cure; some doctors automatically prescribe antibiotics. The overall decline in complications after abortion is due undoubtedly to improved techniques but it is also directly attributable to the increase in early abortions. This increase reflect the assertiveness of adolescent or young women who have chosen not to carry to term an unwanted pregnancy and should be considered as a basic human right of a woman to control her own body and destiny.

Girls who remain in the family after an incestuous rape nearly always manifest hostile-aggressive behavior (55% of the cases); anti-social delinquent behavior (19%); and school problems and school adjustment (57% of the cases)• M Marked erosion in the parent-child relationships was found in 68% of the cases of extreme coercion, and continual contacts of a serious sexual nature. Negative outcome in terms of lasting psychological damage to the child are "highly probable.

This condition rarely improves with time; sadly, the trauma dccpcns as the young victim grows old enough to understand what happened, or as the older one contemplates her family situation. For the most part, the incest victim's reactions are dependent upon her behavioral conditioning by her mother and other members of her family. This kind of mental torment may go on for years, as her father does not report some cases until the daughter becomes pregnant. Unwanted pregnancy added to the impact of fear, anxiety, shame and loss of self-esteem can severely retard the adolescent's emotional development

The Rape Kit, Media and the Courts

Despite new images increasingly presented by the media depicting the "sexual equality" of women and men, the human rights of the rape victim and the intimidating, abusive tactics used against her as an abridgement of the woman's rights, the sexist images of men and women prevail and are frequently used to shore up the sexual prowess of the assailant.

The lower economic social class has never been able to successfully sue to redress a wrong although legal aid has improved personal grievances crimes. Penalties imposed for convicted rapists of upper and middle-class income groups are still usually lighter than those of minority or lower-class groups even if they are accused of the same crime. All too often the morals of economically challenged women and girls are questioned. The defense attorney will ask the victim if she had consensual (willing) sex with anyone in the past 5 days who may also have left behind DNA. Questions of promiscuity must be addressed and the rape kit evidence can be used to determine which DNA was left by a consensual partner and which DNA belongs to the perpetrator.

Even if the victim has not yet decided to report the crime, receiving a forensic medical exam and keeping the evidence safe from damage will improve the chances that the Police can access and test the stored evidence at a later date and Justice can be obtained. The rape kit eliminates or blunts many forms of prejudice.

Various critics have suggested that this situation would be somewhat alleviated if the law would simply define rape as a physical assault and leave out all sexual overtones. Frankly there is anti-woman bias in nearly every case that deals with women and a quick perusal of divorce law finds references to "promiscuous women," "a woman of ill repute," "unchaste women," "his mistress," "adulterous women, 'the mother's indiscretions," etc. Statistics show that when the law is applied to female offenders, women and teenage girls receive sentences for less serious crimes.

A simple assault would be a clear-cut case of violation of individual rights. But with sexist overtones the determination of whether or not those rights legally exist must be first determined by the state's attorney's discretion. The evidence gathered for presentation at the trial as well as the testimony of the victim may not be sufficient to prove a legal right although if the victim has completed the rape kit processes it may be sufficient to prove rape.

Media is the tool, which can and should be used to explore people's roles, to discover alternatives to human conflict and displacement fantasies not rooted in violence. When media's well-paid superstars are blindly followed to their logical antisocial destructive conclusions, intimate relationships and even homes may be disrupted. The individual helplessness of the victim pervades both male and female stereotypes; artificial illusions remain incomplete and unfulfilled.

Many socially aware groups are working toward depicting interpersonal relationships without the crippling psychologies based on infantile sensory needs, the helpless enslavement to flesh and to the power figures that control them. A concern of the women's movement has been to broaden the roles of women presented by all forms of media, including textbooks, to reflect not only the statistics but also the broad diversification of the roles shared by women and men in our technological society.

In order to understand the vital role the rape kit plays in the victim's legal rights it is important to examine the legal process in laywoman's terms. Everyone knows that DNA evidence is collected at a crime scene by trained investigators. Law enforcement and criminal investigators receive special training on the handling of DNA evidence to avoid destruction however DNA evidence can be contaminated.

This is where the rape kit backs up the victim's account of the assault. DNA evidence can be compromised in a number of ways first of all whenever it comes into contact with another person's DNA, There are conditions at the crime scene that are a factor such as if the DNA is exposed to heat, humidity, strains of bacteria and many other environmental conditions.

The rape kit often makes the difference not only in the trial or in only one woman's ordeal. It is the secure handling of the contents of the rape kit that can make certain the evidence necessary to prove rape is not tampered with or damaged. This evidence is preserved and when tested and compared with literally tens of thousands of cold cases involving rape and murder the statistics of crime against women and children change all across America.

The Kit has 16 separate steps to collect evidence. There are detailed instructions for each step that the provider should follow but one important one is the head-to-toe, detailed examination and assessment of the entire body. This assessment has an outline of the female body with places to cite areas of trauma to arms legs head and torso. This assessment also includes the internal examination.

The collection of blood, urine, hair and other body secretion samples may require the testimony of a forensic pathologist or their report. The photographic evidence of injuries such as bruises, cuts and scraped skin are available for selection to be presented by the attorney at trial.

This exam is important because it preserves the DNA evidence is an integral to identifying the perpetrator in a sexual assault case, especially those in which the offender is a stranger. The preservation of DNA evidence is critical in a criminal investigation. The DNA evidence alone can build a strong case to show that a sexual assault occurred. As the rape kits are processed and the DNA samples are tested and matched to criminal data bases the appalling truth is coming to light, men who rape once rape again and again and again.

When the state's attorney determines that a crime has been committed and depending upon the circumstances of the investigation, a preliminary hearing is routine for a felony such as rape. Serving largely as a screening process the evidence contained in the rape kit can be the determining factor against other assault cases competing for priority before a crowded court docket.

A preliminary hearing is conducted without a jury; only the state's attorney and the victim-witness, the suspected offender and his attorney are present to confront the judge. Since this preliminary hearing usually follows within ten days after the suspect is in custody, many victims are still recuperating from trauma or physical injuries suffered by the attack, and so she may or may not be required to testify especially in cases of minors or severely injured victims.

The prosecutor initiates the hearing's proceedings. Presenting as evidence, medical and scientific findings for examination by the judge. Defense experts usually analyze this corroborative material separately and this is where the rape kit really is the victim's best witness. Modern scientific methods of testing DNA and other evidence samples have made the medical evidence contained in the rape kit pertinent in rape cases.

The evidence contained in the rape kit is rapidly changing the statistics and the outcomes of the courts handling of criminal cases involving rape. Semen analysis may be blood-typed and may be found on clothing, fibers, and hair specimens to give a more accurate identification of the suspect or suspects.

Clothing and the photographs of physical injuries taken by the police or at the hospital may be may be displayed in the court as well as photographs displayed that were taken at the scene of the crime.

At this time, pornographic materials found either on the offender's person, in his automobile or apartment is presented as a contributory cause of crime. Pornography has been specifically geared to the tradition-steeped orientation of the male ego as active and the submissive, passive woman as property. The media glamorizes the pornographic themes involving aggression-gratification, which is true in western culture but more apparent in Islamic and near eastern media presentations.

The female role model for an Islamic and many traditional customs conforms to religious or cultural beliefs. The law in those countries is written to reflect the social origins of this injustice and is codified by religious beliefs that are hinged around an assortment of traditional myths and prejudices. In viewing certain international films or cable television programs women activists are struck by the limitations and apparent inequities in the roles of women and men.

Pornography is also being psychologically targeted at women who seek an active role outside the home though in limited quantities. This campaign assumes women's more active roles in their work lives, sexual participation and desire for power and dominance. An example of this strategy backfiring is the counterpart to the magazine Playboy named Playgirl designed to appeal to the sexually liberated woman but which has been found to have a very large male readership.

New definitions are certainly needed, but merely changing laws alone to eliminate the injustices is insufficient— media violence and sexism and the escalating crime rate must be dealt with on a larger scale. Statutes, state constitutions, and legislative interpretations of rape have all been subject to traditional sexist myths. The defense attorney still resorts to portraying his client as the "tough guy" image—a man who resolves personal conflict and social problems through action not words. The woman's behavior indicated she was consenting and he simply acted on her initiative, in other words, the use of violence and criminal behavior was in order. Women disagree.

Once all the evidence has been presented at the preliminary hearing, the state's attorney and the defense attorney discuss the possibility of a plea bargain; the implicit understanding is that the assailant admits some guilt in return for rehabilitation program, a parole or probation. The victim or her parents, has the right to discuss with the prosecutor the possibility of, as well as the full explanation for consideration of a plea bargain.

It is estimated that somewhere between 80 to 90 percent of criminal convictions are the result of the entry of a plea rather than a guilty verdict at the end of a trial, in many district courts "admitting to a finding" relieves the high case load in the courts as well as much of the pressure from the police to dispose of as many cases as possible-4 and also because it is the defense counsel's desire to maintain a good trial record by keeping his clients out of jail.

The state's attorney at this time, if not sooner, confers with the defense attorney and opens up much of his case prior to the actual trial. This is known as "discovery" and means that in order for a trial to take less time and to proceed smoothly (keep adversary momentum and trial delays to a minimum) all information that the prosecutor has accumulated during the course of his and the police's investigation of the rape case will be turned over to the defense attorney. Because of discovery, certain witnesses, including the victim. May be contacted by the offender's attorney although they are not required to make any statements to him outside of the court.

Other people's DNA can influence the investigation leading to confusion of who was present or who participated in the crime. DNA samples are collected from anyone who was known to have been at the crime scene and may include samples form the responding officer and suspects who are family members or friends that can be identified at the scene. If the victim had consensual sex within 72 hours before the assault occurred then that person would be identified and samples requested. All these samples may be admitted as evidence at the trial.

At this time important pieces of evidence may be suppressed because of the inflammatory impact it is assumed the case will have on the jury and on the society. Usually these are cases involving incest or pedophilia moreover, since each attorney's professional advancement depends upon his win-lose trial record, the defense attorney typically tries to convince the prosecutor that his case cannot be won.

When the judge finds "probable cause," the next step in many states is a grand jury hearing where neither the state's attorney with neither the suspect nor his attorney present presents the facts? Under heavy criticism, often denounced as a "rubber stamp" of the judiciary bench, the grand jury consists of 12 to 24 people from the county or community who reflect the public's opinion in the court system.

The grand jury must be able to confirm the judge's determination of "sufficient evidence," by reviewing the evidence and signing off on the decision. The grand jury has the right to deliberate the evidence if the judge acts in any way to appear compromised by the stature in the community of the man or men who are accused. The evidence contained in the rape kit can be the determining factor whether or not the suspected assailant is indicted and the case is authorized to be sent on to the superior court for a trial.

Arraignment generally follows the grand jury's indictment. Here the suspect is given a copy of the charges filed against him, is advised of his constitutional rights and is asked to enter his plea. Each state has own arraignment procedure but the general information given the suspected assailant is that of the Fifth, Sixth, and Fourteenth Amendments to the United States Constitution's Bill of Rights.

When the offender pleads not guilty, the judge will order a trial and set the bail if it has not already been done. It is difficult to understand how a not guilty plea could be entered when the rape kit evidence is a factor. In fact at this stage the DNA evidence may link the offender to a series of rapes or attempted assaults within a geographical area. The rape kit evidence may encourage the offender to plead guilty in which case there will be no trial and the judge will set a date for sentencing.

Under our present legal system it is the responsibility of the judge, the prosecutor, and the defense attorney to confer as to the seriousness of the crime and the amount of sentencing based on the evidence and the offender's past criminal record. Many adult victims and notably parents of child victims have protested the release of certain rapists because of the extreme danger not only to their child but associated with the presence of a pedophile in the community.

Several months may elapse before the actual trial begins due to repeated delays by the defense for the preparation of material, gathering of witnesses and various personal reasons. This can depend upon the type of activity involved in the offense. At the time of the trial the assailant may choose whether to have the case heard before a judge or a jury. His attorney will almost certainly urge him to select a jury trial, particularly if his case is weak.

This strategy is based on the assumption that the victim can be made to look like a willing participant or can be classified by the jury into any number of negative sexist types and her rights discarded along with the charge of rape. It is also an advantage when a past record for criminal behavior is extant whereas a judge could have access to such records, a jury made up of average citizens selected from the voter registration polls, does not.

The socializing influence of the mass media upon the legal professionals and potential jury members may be apparent at this time. Jury members, like most people, are subjected to media indoctrination and all too often accept the media stereotypes as a basis for much of their social interaction. Since mass media communicates the social norms of behavior for both the male and the female, the defense attorney goes along with the program.

The routine is fairly predictable as the defense tries to seat older middle-class men who can be counted on to maintain a sexist double-standard, lower middle-class men who uphold the rugged sports male image and upper middle-class businessmen who travel extensively and whose social profile includes visits to various porn shops or by mail order porn. When selecting female jurors the defense looks for women who dress conformist or are middle-class housewives whose traditional values, reinforced by media, in the belief that these women will predictably condemn the victim and acquit the offender.

During the jury selection process the defense attorney may recommend to the judge to dismiss certain jurors of their civic duty—those whom they consider unfavorable to the defense. These jurors are the ones that the state's attorney has attempt to seat that appear to correspond to the victim's age group as younger working women, female minorities, or those whom he feels will be sympathetic toward the victim.

A trial court must reconstruct from the evidence and the testimony of the victim. At the trial the victim may be asked questions about the testimony given to the police or at the medical facility. The account that was recorded at the time in the "Assault/Abuse History," is usually a very detailed description of the assault. A SANE nurse may elicit responses or clarify facts at the time that are forgotten months later. These critical details may corroborate other evidence or results from the Investigation.

Other evidence left at the crime scene may confirm the clothing you wore during the assault, torn fabric or fibers can place you at the location. The rape exam includes collection of important evidence provided by clothing (especially torn items and undergarments). The victim on the witness stand may be asked fewer questions if her clothing was provided as evidence to be processed with the rape kit. Certain questions regarding provocative attire may be never asked. The rape kit serves as corroboration of the victim's account and the prosecution's next strongest evidence.

It does not matter what you were wearing rape is a violent crime and the clothing you were wearing should be considered as a specimen that can be evidence not for its fashion but for its DNA. If the victim escapes or returns home she may have already changed clothes and may consider washing or destroying that outfit.

Even if the victim has changed clothes she should take the clothes she wore during the assault with you to the medical facility, which will place them in a bag as evidence. Although this is not as effective at trial as presenting to the ER or clinic immediately without changing clothes unless they are too badly damaged.

The trained SANE nurse or doctor who is working with you at the time and who will take various "samples" preserves the critical DNA evidence. Due to trauma or shock most victims do not remember the nurse taking fingernail scrapings, hair samples and oral swabs for evidence collection. At trial this evidence collected under these control conditions and witnessed by a disinterested third party serve to establish the critical difference between your DNA and any other that is found.

Most rape victims have bruises or cuts that may not appear or be noticed until days later. The nurse or doctor at the time you go to the ER or SANE clinic may look at your body using a "Woods Lamp," a fluorescent lamp that allows the practitioner to see evidence that they cannot see with the naked eye. This examination is recorded in the medical record and is part of the rape exam that can be presented at trial to prove rape instead of consensual sex.

Although medical findings indicate that intercourse occurred, this does not necessarily constitute rape. Rape has been disproved despite severe bodily injury or other evidence such as torn clothing and missing buttons can be explained in a number of ways that do not involve rape but the contents of the rape kit do prove rape. Indications of physical trauma in more extreme cases, i.e., the rape of elderly victims or children, have been used to substantiate the state's case even without the victim's testimony but still require the evidence from a rape kit for a conviction.

The various witnesses to the crime, those who saw the suspect with the victim last or saw him near the crime scene perhaps even entering or leaving the apartment or home. Other witnesses are those who were contacted by the victim immediately following the assault. Witnesses to events before or after the assault may be subpoenaed as well—friends, family members, and rape crisis counselors who often arrive at the scene before the police.

Police officers, psychiatric or medical personnel and anyone qualified to evaluate the victim's emotional status in the hospital immediately following the attack are often required to testify. Most police officers give an account of the crime scene and therefore must include a description of the status of the victim but the testimony of the officer is not the sole source of information to determine the crime of rape.

The ER physician at the hospital or the SANE nurse at the campus clinic who conducted the medical examination or any other medical personnel present during the examination may also be subpoenaed. The rape kit is most often the critical piece of evidence along with the medical record submitted to substantiate these professional's testimony. These are the most relied on sources by the jury for understanding the condition of the victim after the assault.

In order to build an orderly sequence of circumstantial evidence corroborating the state's case, the prosecutor asks straightforward questions of the victim on the witness stand. He thereby commences the trial and sets into motion the adversary procedure that characterizes the American court system. His introductory approach is in direct contrast to the techniques employed by the offender's attorney during the cross-examination of the victim.

The mass media presentations of men and women influences public opinion, represented by the jury, and contribute to these legal misunderstandings in terms of the issue of 'consent." Men and women both are expected to imitate the standards of behavior presented by the mass-media enculturation. Today many women are subject to sexual harassment because of pornographic images, a form of unlawful sex discrimination. Prosecutors have thrown out too many cases of harassment of women and girls because they carry the essential plot of numerous Hollywood movies.

By relying on the jury members' exposure to media role models, the legal profession in many states defines its perimeter of inquiry into the sex life of the victim. From TV, magazines and movies the defense attorney's questions originate and from these same sources the answers are already given. How much the witness deviates from them determines in many cases how much her testimony will be believed.

The federal government and most states have passed legislation limiting the kinds of questions that can be asked of the rape victim. Strong restrictions have been written into the law against introducing the victim's prior sex history as admissible evidence. While many states do permit the suspect's attorney to cross examine the victim about certain aspects of her past sex life, it is up to the discretion of the judge to rule where the questions are relevant.

There have been instances when the judge examines witnesses and even has decided to summon witnesses whom neither attorney has called. This blunts the tactics of the defense lawyer who typically tries to prevent the trial judge or jury from correctly evaluating the evidence presented.

An orderly sequence of circumstantial evidence presented to corroborate the victim's testimony by the prosecuting attorney who often asks straightforward questions can be anticipated. It is imperative that there is an earnest attempt on the part of the victim to answer as objectively as possible all the prosecuting attorney's questions. This cooperativeness will be perceived by the jury as honesty and will bring her testimony through the skillful and deceptive techniques of the cross-examiner.

Where some of the facts of a jury trial may be misrepresented by the attorneys or misconstrued by the jury an expert may be called in to interpret these facts. This technique is rarely employed in rape cases unless the victim herself. Her personal attorney or women's advocate works with the prosecutor in the presentation of rape cases in the various counties where active volunteers are present.

By offering the uninformed victim counsel through rape crisis centers, these advocates help with research as well as explain and advise on the entire legal system. This legal aid is generally available through women's centers, which also refer victims to attorneys who will advise on the particulars of legal procedures necessary for the victim herself to assume a more active role in the proceedings of the trial.

Families and the Courts

Despite the statistical facts, a considerable proportion of family violence has been diverted out of the legal process and until recently went underreported as a crime in the society except to be reflected in the rising divorce rate. When such cases come to the family courts they are for one reason or another diverted from the legal process yet these always contain allegations of assault or rape.

If the victim of domestic violence has been physically harmed to the extent that a physical handicap or extreme emotional, psychological trauma renders her incapable of supporting her children, then the husband must be held financially accountable. First the abuse must stop and it is possible for a married woman to obtain a restraining order against her husband and to bring her case to court. Another avenue is through the civil courts where financial reimbursement for damages may be obtained. In some states a divorce may be granted on the evidence contained in the rape kit as proof of cruelty alone.

Like behavior and attitudes, media images change with the generations they are designed to influence. New symbols are adopted for each new generation; much of media articulates these differences and creates suitable fantasies for the masses of individuals it wishes to exploit for profit.

Before making the decision to prosecute a juvenile rape case, the state's attorney carefully determines the strength of his case by considering the supporting physical evidence— the medical report and the evidence found at the scene by police—tattered clothing, bullet or knife wounds, bruises or broken bones, evidence of rape from semen analysis, fingerprints identifying the suspect as being at the scene of the crime, and testimony of other witnesses. Although such corroborating evidence may be available in abundance, it can be overruled by media's extenuating circumstances.

Nearly everyone is influenced by the media images of television and the cinema indeed, social reality is continually being reinterpreted through these models; for example, the media messages and certain forms of music have a derisive and alienating effect upon young persons within the homogeneity of the family unit as well as the society at large. Often the lyrics are antisocial and generational; the product-orientation is specifically geared to the emotional maturity levels of an adolescent.

The ingrained double standard in our society makes legal professionals and juries concerned not so much with determining the assailant's guilt or innocence in the offense. But rather on determining the victim's. When attorneys misconstrue the truth in such cases, the adolescent victims are frequently ruled "too incompetent to testify;"

If her record for junior or senior high school performance is minimal, if she used alcohol or perhaps drugs at any time, or has any type of criminal record whatsoever or simply by virtue of being a young female. The defense attorney will comb the records to produce some evidence that she has engaged in other types of activities not deemed by the justice system to be contributing to the society.

In the case of incest victims past puberty whose identity with feminine role model images—her makeup, hairstyle, skirt lengths and degree of pants* snugness— is seen as all too reflective of her sexuality and whose very appearance is misconstrued as "provocative' or "consensual."

Prosecutors typically refuse to enter such charges of incest if only because of the victim's age. To understand this biased stance by the state's attorney, one must remember that besides being subject to media images, the prosecutor's office is chiefly interested in a good conviction rate that a jury will be asked to prove the attorney will challenge the prosecutor. The general public's impression of teenaged girls is derived from the many tradition bound and sexist role models presented by the media-fabricated the offender's attorney will no doubt select certain characteristics of media sex symbols in an attempt to categorize the victim and her role in the incident.

Incest is rarely brought to trial. On the average Incest reports are not made until the victim grows older or becomes pregnant. Corroborating evidence is difficult to obtain in cases reported weeks, months, or years after the initial offense. When charges are brought they are usually not listed as rape, and they usually only serve to restrict the father's behavior (but most often the child's) or to define the terms of a separation or divorce that will provide economic support for \ the abused child.

There is a great amount of concern expressed by fen family interest groups for the psychological welfare of the very young victim of incest. After much deliberation by the state's attorney and those involved in the criminal justice system it is often decided that the solution to an incest case .s to separate the child from her parents and place her in a foster home or in an institution for homeless girls—but here again it is the girl who becomes the offender and is punished. The reasons given for not carrying these cases to court are many but usually result from the legal professionals' condescending consensus that such a case would inflame the average citizen and cause "immense public discord.

Many victims of crime are finding that a more effective way to pursue justice in our present legal system is through the civil courts. In a criminal incest case other members of the family such as the mother I^ or brothers and sisters refuse to testify in behalf of the victim against their father. In civil cases, pornographic Industries or other commercial concerns can be brought to trial for having contributed to the incestuous behavior of the parent.

Media forms a vital link in the chain of corroborating evidence in an "indecent liberties" case involving children three- to ten-veers of molestation may be accomplished without proving that the crime resulted from exposure to pornographic materials, it can be seen in many instances to contribute to the crime. By virtue of the fact that child porn often involves role-play and scene reenactments are common in rape cases involving children the connection is unmistakable.

In nearly all child rape cases, the defense attorney typically pressures the prosecutor into a plea bargain. Plea bargaining for child molesters results in a reduction of charges against the offender, avoids a lengthy mandatory sentence in favor of release, a rehabilitation program where this program is available (generally only large urban areas), parole or probation status. The generosity of plea bargains can be seen in "Sexually Dangerous Persons" petitions which are considered at this time, if not previously, for possible rehabilitation or 1 reform of the offender.

The testimony of qualified psychiatrists, usually at least three in number, is submitted for the courts consideration along with the evidence presented. Extensive psychiatric treatment may be recommended for both the victim and the molester. Unfortunately, the release of child molesters back into the community has often served to destroy citizens' confidence in the legal system and this is particularly the case for embittered parents of child victims.

Assembly-line production of cases in modern court procedures makes little or no allowance for equal presentation of controversial issues. Even the prosecutor's and the defense attorney's concluding remarks at the trial, and the judge's condescending final instructions to the jury are based on the evidence presented and particular stress is often placed on the degree of corroboration necessary for a conviction in a rape trial. Too often these instructions constitute a biased opinion in the absence of a completed rape kit assessment. When women, mothers, daughters and grandmothers unite to demand a rape kit for every rape the phrase "the charge of rape is easy to make but difficult to prove," will no longer apply.

If the jury has returned a guilty verdict then the court must pronounce sentence although this may occur weeks or months after the verdict has been handed down. During this time the judge may ask for a persistence investigation. This investigation reveals those pieces of evidence not presented to the jury during the course of the adversary attorney trial. In criminal cases, defense attorney and prosecution confer privately in order to reach a compromise on the sentencing of the assailant. Hence, a guilty verdict of rape may result in probation for say a youthful offender, with such conditions as the trauma and suffering of the victim, this can scarcely be considered restitution.

The state's attorney at the sentencing trial must again present the evidence and request a definite sentence for a period of confinement? However, sentencing renegotiations between defense and state's attorneys made prior to this hearing are almost universally always honored. In general, judges show a greater leniency to those offenders who have pleaded guilty to obtain a plea bargain with the court.   Several major sentencing issues along with other suggestions for the movement. Women's advocates have suggested new sentencing brackets that treat rape as an assault and are affecting the revision of many states' rape statistics.

Greater awareness of women's rights violations in the American court system begins in America's law schools. The mandatory participation in a complete rape and sexual assault trial and a thorough knowledge of the evidence procedures with emphasis on the handling of the rape kit is needed. Importance should be attached by the University to student-initiated projects and semester internships funded by federal grants that require not only knowledge of but also participation in court trials and focus on the interaction with litigants in civil and criminal rape cases.

Curricula in law schools would place impetus on student involvement on a full-time basis in the kinds of activities lawyers undertake in civil and criminal cases such as wife beating and rape. The legal profession is most effective as a participant in the realization of society's goals and must reflect the majority of the population. Statistics prove that there are increasingly more women involved in rights issues either racial or gender based.

Their insight on social welfare and personal conflict-resolution mediation should be made available to law students and talks or presentations about these issues stressed in law schools! Students would experience person-to-person contact with women's issues and victims providing a learning environment that promotes women's social issues.

This united front attests to the potential for American Bar Association to provide many constructive criticisms of the judicial process. Books written by these attorneys' judges and other concerned citizens point out the defects and injustices in our legal system, but they almost all agree that change can only be generated by American citizens.

Conclusion

Victims of rape have been put in real physical danger. The way each victim responds to this danger is dependent upon her background and the details of the assault. Universally the victim is in need of support, information and/or assistance in clarifying feelings and options in the immediate aftermath and this is why it is so critical to seek medical care and complete a rape exam. In the initial reaction phase, her friends and family must offer support and guidance to seek care. Studies have shown that immediately following the rape; the victim must cope with intense emotional trauma in addition to physical injuries and emotional pain.

Our bodies and sexual persona are private matters but her assailant has ripped this privacy from the rape victim. She may be too embarrassed to discuss the physical details of the rape to anyone she knows and doesn't know enough about the procedure to undergo a medical exam. Too many rapes go unreported out of fear and ignorance and the statistics will not go down until women realize they must do the right thing and get checked out and tested for disease.

Shock will convince even an intelligent woman to attempt a return to her normal routines, avoiding all attempts to recognize consciously that a rape has occurred. Many victims of date rape drugs exhibit a decreased appetite and unexplained stomach pains or nausea. The drugs suppressed the mental awareness of the rape incident, and questions such as "How have you been sleeping or you seem disturbed?" She may have insomnia or nightmares that involve violent or frightening themes that resemble the rape experience or flashbacks in which she feels trapped and unable to escape. These feelings must be addressed no matter how well she knew her assailant. Some women express anger once the rape surfaces and it is this emotion, which is the healthiest response for a victim to express; she has been attacked and humiliated she has a right to be angry.

Even if drugs were not involved the victim may continue with her life exactly as it was before the rape in an attempt to deny it to her and to others. Emotional problems develop and the victim may be irritated with friends of both sexes and become cautious in all her relationships. The victim may spend months painfully recounting the rape as she becomes aware of the necessity to release her negative feelings. If she knew her attacker she may attempt to rationalize and classify the rapist and avoid that type of man in the future.

Some victims examine every thought, gesture, or movement to see what could have caused the attack. This intense self-examination is rarely is productive and only heightens her awareness of her perceived vulnerability. Attempting to reestablish her feeling of security by analyzing how the attack came about the adult victim can be more in control of its future occurrence, giving her more confidence. After the attack many women experience a depression that reaches such a low point that the emotions must be confronted in order to finally resolve them and go on living with herself.

In the instance of a recent assault, many victims will be disoriented and confused. Having been placed in a powerless situation or feels powerless to do anything; this includes her ability to get in touch with her own feelings and work from there. When a rape victim is in trauma, it is imperative that she is able to talk about her feelings to an experienced professional. At this time a supportive, understanding individual can be essential to encourage and assist her to go to the nearest SANE clinic or hospital for care.

Anger at the assailant has ranged from vague thoughts to talk of "getting back" at the rapist. Fathers, brothers and husbands of victims have felt helpless in not knowing "what to do about" the situation or "how to help" the victim. They have felt frustrated because they cannot change what happened. Husbands, male lovers and friends have also mentioned feeling concern about how the victim will relate to them after the rape. Some men feel unsure of how to approach the victim and fear rejection. Many male friends and family members are genuinely concerned about the victim but strong emotions and stereotypic attitudes may override their ability to be humanely supportive.

At a SANE (Sexual Assault Nurse Examiner) staffed clinic or hospital professionals are trained in dealing with the victim encouraging her to express her feelings and by listening to her at this critical time she is calmed and able to accept those family members genuinely showing understanding. SANE trained professionals provide support to the friend, parent, family member, or other person significant to the victim regardless of sex and can provide instructions on how to provide needed supportive contact with the child, adolescent, adult or elderly woman who is in crisis.

When asking the victim questions, open-ended ones are most effective because these questions cannot be answered with simple yes or no responses. Statements such as "Can you describe those feelings" or "I'm listening, you can go ahead" are examples of open invitations to talk. It is essential that the victim explain what happened their own words first and not listen to what others heard her say about the attack. This is necessary for evidence collection and it is a good way to let her know she is being understood.

The supportive individual may share the victim's verbal and non-verbal feelings and emotions but must limit how they share their perceptions with her to only a reflection of feelings. The victim must have self-expression but needs to get back in control of her in order to provide the statement of events. Phrases like "It seems as though you're calmer now than you were before, is that so?" can be helpful to the victim in perceiving her own reactions and getting in touch with herself.

The SANE nurse is familiar with various types of trauma, alternative situations and the institutional set-up through which a rape victim may find healing. This valuable resource is free and should be sought out as soon as possible after an assault. The SANE nurse may work with crisis counselors and social workers who have a list of services that are available and can present them to the victim in a calming manner by asking "Do any of these options feel comfortable to you?" which allows the victim to choose her own solutions. This is critical if the adult, adolescent or child is to regain her own decision-making power and faith in herself going forward. It is her life and her decisions.

Women are aware of their rights and are refusing to be victimized. Women are coming together in groups to make the statistics about rape known and they are making a difference. Changes in awareness and in the practices in our society only happen as people make their voices heard not only for themselves, but also for the children, our future young women. America is committed to the goal of human rights, and as American women who constitute more than half of the population; we feel very strongly that rape is a violation of human rights.

www.ingramcontent.com/pod-product-compliance
Lightning Source LLC
Chambersburg PA
CBHW070356290526
45790CB00004B/1517